Breathe in...
Feel the breath.
Breathe out...
Feel the breath.
This is breath awareness,
A way to calmness, focus, and joy.

CALM FOCUS JOY

The Power of Breath Awareness

A Practical Guide for Adults and Children

HEIDI THOMPSON

COLDSTREAM BOOKS

Disclaimer: This book is sold with the understanding that the author is not engaged to render any type of professional advice and is not intended as a substitute for the medical advice of physicians. No warranties or guarantees are expressed or implied by the author and the author shall not be liable for any physical, psychological, emotional, or financial damage of any kind. The book's content, instructions, suggestions for practice, and theoretical ideas are the sole expression and opinion of the author based on knowledge derived from personal experience. The author and publisher's views and rights are the same: You are responsible for your own choices, actions, and results.

Author: Heidi Thompson
Design: Heidi Thompson (www.heidithompson.ca)
Primary Editor: Heather Hollingworth
Contributing Editors: Angela Gibbs-Peart, Carmen Thompson, Paul Lima
Calm Focus Joy Website (www.calmfocusjoy.com)

Published by: COLDSTREAM BOOKS
9905 Coldstream Creek Road, Coldstream
British Columbia, Canada V1B 1C8

First Edition copyright © 2012 by Heidi Thompson

Library and Archives Canada Cataloguing in Publication
Thompson, Heidi, 1956-

Calm focus joy: the power of breath awareness : a practical guide for adults and children / Heidi Thompson.

ISBN 978-0-9698147-4-0 (Paperback)

1. Attention. 2. Attention in children. 3. Breathing exercises. 4. Meditation—Therapeutic use. I. Title.

LB1065.T56 2011 153.1'532 C2011-901585-4

ACKNOWLEDGEMENTS

I thank Ted for his loving support. I am deeply grateful for my teachers, especially Goenkaji. I thank Heather, Carmen, Angela, and Paul for their heartfelt editing. I thank my mother for raising me to be open-minded. I thank Kathleen, Peter, and all my dear friends for their encouragement. May you all share my happiness.

CONTENTS

Ten-step Mindmastery Program

PREFACE

CALM FOCUS JOY offers a comprehensive program for teaching *breath awareness* to adults and children. Breath awareness is a simple, yet effective exercise that improves focus and reduces stress. It is easy to learn and positive results can be experienced immediately.

Throughout the 5000 years that breath awareness has been in existence, it has reportedly helped millions of people live healthier and happier lives. In the past decade, in fact, researchers have established that breath awareness and other similar focusing techniques strengthen areas of the brain that are responsible for self-regulation, learning, memory, cognition, emotion, and empathy. In addition, other studies confirm that breath awareness boosts the immune system, reduces anxiety, and relieves depression. Not only can breath awareness be used as a preventative measure, therefore, but it can also be used as a remedy for many modern-day maladies.

Whether a beginner, or one seasoned in the art of meditation, Calm Focus Joy's step-by-step program provides in-depth instructions to successfully learn and practice breath awareness. Supporting each practical lesson, a theoretical framework consisting of stories, basic instructions, teacher tips, and suggestions for practice is given. Subsequent chapters outline current research, questions and answers, and facilitation guidelines to provide all that is needed to organize and to teach breath awareness in one's home, classroom, or community.

Over the years, I have taught a breath awareness program called *Mindmastery* to children of all ages and abilities. Almost every child who participated enjoyed learning the exercise and often made comments such as, "Mindmastery was hard, but I want to continue." Encouraged by consistently positive outcomes and the ease of implementing programs into classrooms, I compiled my lessons, stories, and student instructions into a teaching manual, which has now evolved into this book.

The world's most valuable resource is the human mind. Let us do everything within our power to protect, nurture, and develop this precious commodity. We know that happiness and health are achievable through the cultivation of calmness, focus, and joy; therefore, by establishing peace and happiness within, and empowering children in the same way, we will have taken a giant step in transforming our world into a better place.

THE POWER OF BREATH AWARENESS

*Just as pure water restores physical health, pure
breath awareness restores the mind's health.*

The mind is a flexible, living organism with an amazing ability to re-shape itself with every experience it encounters. When we understand how experience influences the mind and changes the brain, we acquire the knowledge to cultivate joy, peace, and wisdom.

A conscious and developed mind is like a powerful jet that can take you to virtually any desired destination. However, if you are unable to focus, the mind remains as ineffective as an aircraft without a pilot. No matter how much you want to get somewhere, lack of focus will always lead you astray. The very act of focusing attention harnesses the mind's incredible power, a power that will help you to achieve your innermost wish. If your goal is to be healthy and happy, developing focus is the essential first step.

Many exercises increase focus; however, not all concentration-training techniques result in the cultivation of mental calm, happiness, and intelligent insight. To nurture these qualities, focus training requires three essential things. First, it should be practiced repeatedly with sufficient intensity to develop the areas of the brain responsible for happiness and empathy. Second, it should heal the root cause of restlessness and dissatisfaction to ensure lasting results. Third, it should facilitate experience that awakens consciousness, self-knowledge, and wisdom. If you reshape the brain into a more intelligent and capable instrument, heal discontent at its source, and grow self-aware, you will enjoy a life abundantly filled with health, joy, and wisdom.

This book teaches a simple technique that can transform you into a more calm, focused, and happy person—not just temporarily, but for the rest of your life! The lessons found in each chapter teach *breath awareness*—a concentration strengthening exercise that develops mental faculties including memory, attention, perception, intuition, and intellect. Breath awareness also promotes brain development, physical health, and provides immediate and long-term relief from unhappy physiological, emotional, and psychological states. It not only calms the mind's surface, it also changes the mind at its deeper levels. Breath awareness can heal the very cause of disease and discontent. Just as physical health is restored with exercise and nutrition, the mind can be healed with breath awareness.

The mind is our greatest gift, our most valuable faculty. Mind is the instrument that lets us experience joy, sense beauty, and feel love. It is the origin of intelligence, creativity, inspiration, thoughts, dreams, and imagination. If the mind is dull or delusional it becomes the source of much misery. If our goal is to achieve joy and peace, we must find a way to eliminate the harmful mental conditioning that keeps us from being happy. Breath awareness provides a way to achieve this goal.

Breath awareness has been used to relieve physical, mental, and emotional suffering, and to awaken self-knowledge for over 2,500 years. The original technique has been preserved in its purity and passed down from teacher to student. During the past fifty years it has gained popularity, especially in the West, and is currently being practiced by millions of people around the world. Its original Pali name is *anapana-sati*, which translated means *breathing in and breathing out with awareness.*

Breath awareness works for anyone, regardless of age, race, politics, culture, or religion. As it is non-dogmatic or religious, it does not conflict or undermine a person's beliefs, rituals, or practices. Breath awareness is traditionally taught freely to any person who wants to learn and costs nothing more than a little time each day to perform. Of the many reasons that people choose breath awareness over other mind-strengthening exercises, the first and foremost reason is that *it works*.

People enjoy breath awareness for many reasons. Not only is it easy to learn, it produces immediate results rather than taking days, weeks, or months to affect change. Just a few minutes of breath awareness can calm agitation, settle distress, and rejuvenate a weary mind. Breath awareness is also convenient. As the object of focus is breath, it can be practiced anytime, anywhere. Breath is with you day and night and you can never forget it at home when you go on vacation!

Many people use breath awareness to manage serious conditions such as depression, ADHD, obsessive-compulsive behavior, and anxiety. For some, breath awareness helps to lower blood pressure, minimize chronic fatigue, and balance mood swings. It can be helpful for those trying to overcome a drug or alcohol addiction, and its calming effect can provide solace to those suffering from the loss of a loved one or from other trauma.

Breath awareness provides a way to examine one's mind/body phenomenon. Some psychologists, scientists, doctors, and lay people use the technique to gain experiential knowledge about how the human mind works. Through actual experience, they learn about mental conditioning, habit responses, instincts, brain processes, attention, and memory. They gain understanding of how thoughts can trigger the brain to produce hormones, neurotransmitters, and other biochemistry, which in turn affect one's emotions and physiology.

Although breath awareness is neither a religion nor a belief, many people use it for meditation and spiritual development. Practicing not only calms and purifies the mind, it can also evoke profound spiritual experience. For centuries, breath awareness has been a way to awaken self-knowledge, instill compassion, and define one's purpose. It dissolves delusional thinking and allows one to see reality as it really is; not how one thinks or believes it to be. Breath awareness transports a person to his or her peaceful center—to that safe refuge found within.

Perhaps you are reading this book as a tool to help reduce stress rather than seeking something profound or spiritual. Even if you are not looking for enlightening knowledge, when you practice breath awareness, you will invariably experience flashes of insight. Awakening of consciousness happens to anyone who works seriously. Even young children realize more self-awareness and knowledge.

Because breath awareness offers so many benefits, both for adults and children, it is certainly a valuable skill to acquire. The purpose of this book is to present an easy-to-follow method that teaches this simple yet powerful technique so that optimum results can be achieved.

The Goal of Focus Training
Breath awareness is a powerful tool that one must learn to practice properly. If not practiced in the right manner, strong, focused concentration could lead a person in an unwholesome direction. Merely developing the ability to concentrate well does not guarantee happiness or peace. To achieve long term, positive benefits, breath awareness incorporates three essential components—*wholesome conduct, awakening insight*, and *sharing goodwill*. The first component of breath awareness, wholesome conduct, refers to how a person lives, behaves, thinks, speaks, and acts. It means living without harming anyone, including oneself. Unwholesome actions, like taking intoxicants, stealing, killing,

or lying can agitate the mind. A person whose mind is severely agitated will find practicing breath awareness very difficult.

Living a wholesome life enhances the development of a person's focus and inner peace. To grow physically healthy, you have to keep working at it by eating well and exercising. The same principle applies to mental health. You need to live a wholesome life and practice mind-strengthening exercises. Living in a wholesome way will help you progress steadily toward your goals of calm, focus and joy. By not harming yourself or others your mind will become more pure and you will have fewer personal obstacles to overcome. When your mind is pure, you will enjoy real happiness.

Focus training should also lead to more self-knowledge. The second component of breath awareness, awakening insight, fulfills this requirement. When you perform breath awareness you learn a great deal about your mind and how it influences your physical body and feelings. When you experience these connections and further investigate your body at its deeper levels of sensation, instinct, mental processes, and body chemistry, you become more self-aware.

Focus training should also foster love and kindness and that is why breath awareness incorporates a third component, sharing goodwill. If concentration exercises were performed only to be self-serving they would not lead to real happiness, nor would the result benefit the rest of humanity. When focus is used for selfish reasons the outcome might cause others to suffer. But if what you do to help yourself in turn helps others, you will solve this problem. To ensure positive outcomes for both you and the rest of the world, breath awareness incorporates the practice of sharing goodwill. Sharing goodwill is the act of sending out a compassionate wish for all beings to share your happiness and peace.

Those who practice breath awareness, while leading a wholesome life, grow in empathy, understanding, and generosity. With an abundance of goodness overflowing from within, sharing happens naturally. When you share your virtues, you benefit a hundredfold. Not only do you benefit by feeling healthier and happier, but your kind volition helps your family, friends, community, and the world.

Work Worth Doing

Breath awareness requires work, and to experience its transformative effect, perseverance, discipline, and patience are needed. Mastering a distracted, restless mind is difficult for anyone. Nevertheless, those who work diligently enjoy wonderful rewards.

One desirable quality you will cultivate is *equanimity*. Equanimity is a person's ability to observe calmly what he or she is experiencing, whether pleasant or unpleasant, while not generating craving or aversion. Equanimity gives a person the power and wisdom to refrain from wanting, either wanting pain to disappear or wanting pleasure to continue. Wanting indicates attachment and dissatisfaction, and is usually the root cause of suffering.

Practicing breath awareness causes you to experience the impermanent nature of your physical and mental structure. This leads to realizing a fundamental truth that frees you from perpetually clinging, craving, and wanting. While seeing the transience of your thoughts and experiencing the changing characteristics of body sensations, you inevitably comprehend why attachment to ever-transforming phenomenon is futile. Attachment to that which is impermanent can only lead to disappointment and depression; while equanimity lets you embrace change with a peaceful mind.

Although breath awareness requires work, positive results are usually experienced after the first session. When you practice regularly and lengthen your sitting times, transformation is obvious. Not only is your disposition more cheerful but your days also unfold more positively. As you continue, deep-rooted and unhealthy conditioning like anger or depression dissolves. When the root causes of your unhappiness are gone, you feel great!

Another desirable quality that breath awareness develops is *mindmastery*. Mindmastery is a quality and state of mind that is self-disciplined and self-aware. A person possessing mindmastery understands how the mind works, is proactive rather than reactive, and is effectual in all areas of life. Being the master of one's mind is freedom; the kind of freedom that you can create within yourself.

Helping You Help Others

This book serves two purposes. One, it helps you to learn the breath awareness technique. Two, it mentors you in becoming a teacher for children. You can begin learning the technique on your own by following the ten *Your Practice* sessions found at the start of each chapter. Simply read the guidelines, perform the exercise, and then reflect on the questions posed in *Check-in* at the end of the chapter.

The lessons become progressively demanding, but you may take as long as you like to work through the ten steps. It might take a couple of weeks to complete the entire program or it might take a few months. There is no advantage to rushing or jumping ahead; real transformation takes time. With experience, you will become confident in practicing the technique and will notice positive transformation in yourself. Three qualities that become increasingly apparent are selflessness, empathy, and compassion. When this happens, you may feel compelled to help children learn this helpful technique.

To assist in this noble mission, Calm Focus Joy provides virtually everything you will need to facilitate a Mindmastery program and teach young people how to do breath awareness. Each chapter-step includes Teacher Tips, which explain the technique, read-aloud instructions followed by a guided breath awareness session for children, a fun story, and topics that can be used for the children's journal writing. Altogether, this information provides you with a comprehensive teaching manual that can be used as is or adopted to your special circumstances or age groups.

When inspired and ready to organize and teach your own Mindmastery program, more helpful guidelines can be found in the following chapters: *You, the Teacher, Facilitating a Mindmastery Program, Sample Application Forms, Student and Teacher Experience* and *Questions and Answers.*

May your journey begin with determination and inspiration and be rewarded with self-knowledge, peace, wisdom, and happiness.

MINDMASTERY

Mastering others is strength. Mastering yourself is true power.
—Tao Te Ching

Breath awareness develops *mindmastery*. Mindmastery is a word that describes an intelligent aptitude cultivated through mind purification, self-knowledge, and wisdom. Mindmastery is an unconditioned state of mind that is free from attachment, ignorance, and delusion. A person who develops mindmastery is composed, disciplined, and compassionate. Such a person has power over their conscious and unconscious behavior and is no longer controlled by instincts, habits, or conditioning.

We are all creations of our conditioning. Even while we were embryos in our mothers' wombs our genetic predispositions, evolved over thousands of years, predetermined many of our instincts, traits, and behaviors. During our formative childhood, our thinking, behaviors, emotional responses, perceptions, beliefs, and even our brains' physiology were further shaped and conditioned by our interaction with social and environmental circumstances. Through repeating certain behaviors and thoughts, we encouraged the creation of fixed neural circuitry in particular areas of the brain, which again shaped our behaviors, skills, and habits.

Now as adults, we behave, feel, relate, speak, react, and think according to how our brains have developed and how our minds have been conditioned. But it doesn't stop here. Our flexible brains continue reshaping their neural circuitry with each new experience. Our brains continue to respond, react, adapt, and change according to internal and external sensory information and stimuli. Studies now show, that even in old age, our brains continue to have the capacity to change, expand, evolve, and recreate who we are, how we think, and how we behave.

Conditioning is generally the root cause of our psychological, physiological, or societal problems. Every aspect of our lives is governed by some degree of conditioning. Survival instincts, behaviors, what we eat, how we educate ourselves, establish relationships, formulate philosophies, prioritize our needs, and even feelings of patriotism or religion are influenced by conditioned thinking. Conditioning does help establish order and workability for a society, but it can also cause people to justify their behavior regardless of the consequences; perpetuate racism, suppressing and exploiting others, or destroying the environment for financial gain. Conditioned actions combined with a lack of awareness, can lead to serious consequences to our health and happiness, and to the well-being of others.

External forces are not the only things responsible for shaping who we are. All on our own, we have systematically conditioned ourselves. How we think, act, and speak today often mimics the behaviors we developed as a child in our innocent attempt to secure survival and our parents' love. What we said or did to obtain praise, rewards, love, attention, and protection in the past oftentimes become ingrained behaviors. Unfortunately, performing these behaviors as an adult may not produce the sought after results.

If you are having difficulties in life with your relationships, work, or self-esteem, or notice that problems keep repeating themselves, check to see if you are behaving in ways similar to when you were a child. If the behavior worked in childhood, your conditioned mind will compel you to use the same tactics in adulthood. Virtually nothing that we say, do, or think is independent of some form of conditioning; hence, we remain psychologically trapped in our behavioral patterns and ingrained habit responses.

Generally, we are not overly concerned about our conditioning as long as our conduct, speech, mannerisms, and customs are accepted or condoned by our society, family, friends, and partners. However, when we start to suffer mentally, physically, or spiritually from our behavior, we may want to change our ways, even if we go against what others want for us. Liberating ourselves from ingrained, subconscious, controlling forces is extremely difficult. Nevertheless, if we become independent of our conditioning, we will experience abundant joy and freedom.

Mindmastery is a Quality
The concept of mindmastery is sometimes misconstrued. Some argue that humans should not attempt to control their natural instincts and responses. They believe that controlling creative impulsiveness stifles spontaneity and self-expression. Others argue that mastering the mind implies imposing control against one's will. Mindmastery, however, is exactly the opposite because mental self-discipline is not achieved through forceful suppression of one's instincts. Rather, mindmastery is a state that comes about when a person's mind is free from condition-

ing; when a person sees clearly, understands thoroughly, and knows deeply.

Developing mindmastery actually causes more spontaneity and creativity. When the mind is pure and free, whatever one says or does will be wholesome. An artist who has developed a pure mind is spontaneous in the execution of his or her craft. The resulting artistic expression reflects the harmonious qualities of the artist's mind.

Self-concept, or ego, is also a creation of our conditioning. When eradicating old conditioning, therefore, we might feel threatened that our self-identity is also being erased. This fear of change makes us cling to our beliefs, defending and protecting them rather than experiencing true freedom.

Many Names, One Technique

The ten breath awareness lessons presented in this book are altogether called the *Mindmastery Program.* When you teach breath awareness to children, you may call your program by another name. A few titles include Sensory Awareness, Anapana, Focus Building, Attention Development, Mental Mastery, Mindfulness, or Breathing Meditation.

When you choose the name, it is better not to use a title that promises a specific outcome, for example "The ADHD Cure". Promising a result, may cause a student to become preoccupied with relieving the ailment, rather than focusing on the breath. Although, breath awareness does, in fact, prevent and cure some conditions, if seeking a remedy becomes the object of focus, the technique's effect will be compromised. This is because the student may, instead of objectively observing the breath, be preoccupied with thoughts of curing an undesirable condition. If the student practices breath awareness, but is continually wanting to fix a problem, this wanting would counteract the goal of developing equanimity. Over the years, I have found that the broad term *mindmastery* fittingly describes the purpose and goal of learning breath awareness. It is also a word enjoyed by younger children because it encapsulates the idea of becoming one's own master and gaining self-empowerment.

Regardless of the different ways to describe the technique or call the program, being mindful of the incoming and outgoing breath as a way to strengthen concentration and calm the mind has been around for a long time. The earliest recorded writings about the power of breath were the Indian Vedas (book of sacred knowledge) dating back 5000 years. Breath awareness is by no means a modern therapy or newly invented program. Countless people in the past practiced breath aware-ness, and millions are practicing today.

One of the better-known breath awareness techniques is *anapana-sati* or *anapana*, which translated means *to breathe in and breathe out with awareness.* During the 11th century B.C., anapana was rediscovered and taught by Gautama the Buddha. The enlightened teacher found it a helpful exercise to prepare his disciples and monks for the more rigor-ous sensation awareness technique called *vipassana*. Vipassana means *to see reality as it is* or *to see with discernment.* Anapana and vipassana were practiced widely both in north and south Asia for hundreds of years before spreading outside of India and Asia. Today you will find vipas-sana and anapana taught in almost every country in the world.

The Transformation

When a person first practices breath awareness it may seem difficult or unnatural. It takes considerable self-discipline and motivation to get past first base. In fact, both adults and children might work for several weeks before they can sit for the suggested times set out in the Mind-mastery Program. However, with perseverance, sitting becomes easier and the benefits experienced will inspire and motivate you to continue. You will feel calmer, less restless, and more patient. You may find that depression, anxiety, and hopelessness diminish. Your mental energy, creativity, and ability to focus will be noticeably enhanced. You may react less severely to what people say or do, you may listen with more empathy, you may refrain from judging others, and you may be more thoughtful when voicing your opinions.

The more you practice breath awareness, the more you gain mastery over your chaotic, scattered, sensation-triggering thoughts. Once you have mental mastery you can harness your mind's instinctive, and often blind responses to life events. Blind reaction is a conditioned response and is the primary contributing factor when it comes to hurting others or yourself. You never intentionally set out to hurt others, nevertheless if you hear yourself saying, *but I didn't mean to do it,* you have probably had first-hand experience with blind reaction. Mastering our reactive habit-mind is one of the most valuable skills we can acquire. Mindmas-tery and self-discipline give us power to choose how we behave, speak, and act. Maybe we could go as far as to say that one who masters reac-tions, masters one's destiny.

AWAKENING INSIGHT

*Self-observation brings man to the realization of the necessity of self-change.
And in observing himself, a man notices that self-observation itself brings
about certain changes in his inner processes. He begins to understand that
self-observation is an instrument of self-change, a means of awakening.*
—George Gurdjieff

Breath awareness is unique in that it awakens insight and leads a person to self-knowledge and wisdom. *Awakening insight* is an essential component of this particular technique, although insight and wisdom will not become apparent from reading the information in this book. Rather, those bright flashes of clarity simply happen while practicing breath awareness.

Breath awareness provides a way to investigate the mind/body phenomenon, enabling a person to examine how the mind works and how emotion, feeling, and experience are all rooted in bodily sensations. Your examination will allow you to differentiate how the mind perceives a stimulus, judges it, instinctively reacts, stores the memory, and ultimately creates conditioning. You will come to know how thought, feeling, emotion, and sensation are co-dependent.

Through actual experience, you will learn how bodily sensations are the root cause of most behavior, and are responsible for developing habits and addictions. You will also experience the surfacing of unconscious and suppressed mind states, and learn how to transform them.

Should you find that breath awareness is not providing insightful experiences, you might be practicing incorrectly for either of two common reasons. First, you may be spending the hour of practice engrossed in thought. If the mind stays preoccupied intellectually, it cannot stay connected with feeling. Your attention cannot be two places at once; it is either feeling or thinking. While doing breath awareness, the secret is to stay focused on feeling.

A second reason may be that your mind is overly agitated. What you think, say, or do outside of breath awareness practice will directly affect your capacity to focus. If you have performed an unwholesome action, indulged in an intoxicant, or hurt someone, your mind will be disturbed. A restless mind cannot focus well and will lack sufficient stillness and intensity to penetrate the deeper levels of the unconscious. It is only when you work at these deeper levels that you experience profound transformation and mind purification.

Using Focus to Awaken Insight

Focus is a powerful tool—a force that helps us to accomplish countless goals. Ideally, humans would apply focus to achieve healthy, life-sustaining, and humanitarian goals. As it is, our world is not so ideal and some people use focus for selfish or destructive purposes. Whether intentional or not, focus is often used to exploit people, organize warfare, mastermind crime, or misuse our planet. However, just because the world is less than ideal, we can still take personal responsibility for our actions and choose to pursue a constructive, worthwhile goal.

Unfortunately, even if we take responsibility for our actions and focus on a worthy goal we are still susceptible to stress, depression, and ill health. Focus alone cannot guarantee happiness or inner peace. Professors, scientists, doctors, politicians, actors, artists, and athletes may focus and excel in their careers only to fall victim to a weakness or an addiction. Despite excellent focus, if a person compromises ethical integrity or succumbs to some form of obsessive behavior, unhappiness can result.

The best assurance that breath awareness focus training leads to knowledge, wisdom, and joy, comes from establishing an ethical foundation within yourself. For this reason, breath awareness goes hand in hand with *wholesome conduct*, which means *to live, speak, and act in a way that does not harm others or oneself*. It is fundamental to the technique. Without wholesome conduct, breath awareness would not yield the same results. Wholesome conduct guarantees that wherever you apply your focus, the outcome will be healthy.

Experiential Knowledge

We often assume that we know something after reading information. Reading provides an intellectual understanding of a subject; facts, theories, and concepts inform us so we can communicate with each other, make decisions, and function in the world. Even so, this kind of intellectual knowledge is limited and has minimal effect when it comes to transforming ingrained conditioning, knowing ourselves, or creating happiness.

Take swimming for example. You can read books on how to swim. You can study the physics of floatation. You can observe professional swimmers and listen to instructors explain stroke techniques. All this knowledge might make you believe that you know how to swim. Nevertheless, apparent knowledge says nothing about whether you can actually swim. Only after you plunge into water, experience a sinking feeling, kick your feet, swing your arms, and propel ahead, can you say, *Yes, I know how to swim*. You know how to swim by doing it. The same principle applies to breath awareness. Even if you read this book a dozen times and memorize its entire contents, you still will not be able to do breath awareness. You only know breath awareness by *doing it*.

Uprooting Negative Seeds

While practicing breath awareness you will learn, through your own experience, about complex psychological processes relating to your conscious and unconscious mind. Children, however, might not comprehend what is happening to them while practicing. To help them intellectually understand their experiences, each step includes simple analogies to clarify how breath awareness works.

One frequently used illustration compares the contents of our unconscious mind, including all its memories, inherited psychological and physiological traits, conditioned behaviors, to a mind-garden filled with thousands of seeds. These seeds lay buried deep within our subconscious. Since birth, we have accumulated countless memory-seeds and although they are not visible to our conscious mind, they exist and affect how we feel. Each seed possesses a different quality and characteristic. Some have wholesome, positive traits while others are destructive to our emotional or psychological well-being. At any time, a seed can be watered by life's circumstances or by our thoughts or actions, and start to sprout. When a memory-seed manifests, it creates a thought and a corresponding sensation, which the conscious mind becomes aware of.

Each memory-seed is one unit comprising two components: a conceptualized image, thought, or word and a sensation, emotion, or feeling. The image might be something that we saw or imagined; the word or concept might be something we heard or thought up. The connecting sensation might be pain, pleasure, pressure, tingling, numbness or heaviness; the feeling or emotion could be happiness, sadness, fear, or resent.

To understand the image/word/sensation/feeling unit, imagine a happy incident in your past. Think of your first love or infatuation. Immediately, a picture of a person arises in your mind or you hear his or her words, *I love you*. The image or words evoke a sensation. Your heart swells; you feel pleasant. Even though the romantic incident might have occurred years ago, your memory still evokes a loving sensation. Now imagine a painful event. Perhaps, your elementary teacher embarrassed you in front of your class. The unpleasant image of your teacher appears in your mind along with any criticizing words she might have spoken. Your stomach tightens; your heart pounds. Years after the experience, the teacher's horrible image and the sensations of pain and shame are still connected.

Your memory bank comprises millions of these complex memory-seeds that lay dormant in your subconscious until something provokes them to surface in your conscious mind. Some memory-seeds are harmless, while others cause ongoing stress.

When speaking of deep-rooted psychological problems we are often referring to suppressed memories that simmer below the surface and cause us to feel uneasy, depressed, or unhappy. Practicing breath awareness helps to uproot these invisible, suppressed memories making them tangible and easier to work with. Unlike psychotherapy or self-analysis, though, you will not try to understand your condition by imagining or remembering what happened. You actually refrain from such intellectual, conceptual psychoanalysis. Rather, in breath awareness, you will be keeping your attention fixed on feeling sensations. Your sensations will no doubt be connected to a memory, but you will not concern yourself with this memory. The key will be to stay exclusively focused on *feeling* the breath—its warm or cool sensation as it passes over the skin, and acknowledging, but not dwelling on imagined past or future events.

Breath awareness is like an operation of the mind, whereby you facilitate toxic memories to surface and then systematically remove them. This operation helps transform and thus eliminate unhealthy, repressed memory-seeds until your mind is uncontaminated. When destructive memories dissipate, they can longer cause stress, depression, or anger and you feel happier. Breath awareness helps transform and dissolve conditioned mind states—where fear becomes understanding; anger becomes forgiveness; resentment becomes love.

Performing breath awareness is straightforward. It involves focusing on the *touch* of respiration, which in turn calms the mind. When the

mind is calm, memories surface into the conscious mind and simultaneously cause a bodily sensation.

When memories surface, the mind's eye then sees an image or starts
thinking about an idea. Along with this image or idea, you feel a sensation or emotion. Sometimes the image appears before the feeling becomes apparent. Sometimes the feeling emerges, and then an image or
idea forms. When we are not attentive, it may appear as though the image or thought, and sensation or feeling is one thing arising simultaneously. Closer examination reveals that they are two separate events.

In breath awareness, we continually fix our attention on the feeling
event—the sensation of breath on the skin. The more our attention stays
engaged with feeling, the fewer thoughts, ideas, concepts, or mental
images manifest in our mind. When we practice breath awareness, the
goal is to separate the sensation from its mental image. Once they are
two separate entities, the sensation can be observed objectively for what
it is, rather than be associated with a memory, concept, or imagined
event. For example, the physical sensations of sadness such as heaviness, numbness, or pain can be examined without thinking about what
may have caused the feeling. With discriminating focus we can observe
the characteristics of the sensation without reacting to it or conjuring up
mental images that may distract us from feeling our breath. A tangible
sensation provides us with something real to work with. We feel the
breath's soft, tingly, warm, or cool touch on the skin, which is real experience. We are not imagining these sensations, nor are we creating a
conceptualization of them.

Often, when we concentrate exclusively on feeling the breath, sensations elsewhere in the body intensify. These sensations may be ones of
strain, throbbing, pressure, agitation, frustration, sadness, pain, restlessness, boredom, or uneasiness. When doing breath awareness properly, you would refrain from reacting to these aches, pains, and
emotional states. You would try not to move, get up, or let your mind
start wandering, thinking, or imagining. By staying focused only on
feeling breath, the discomfort might intensify and continue for a while,
but eventually it diminishes. The more you can weaken your habit-
responses, the more your habits lose their control over you.

As you can see, non-reactive observation of sensation is the key to
eradicating unhealthy habits. Modifying our habit-response to pain,
frustration, fear, or anger through objective observation eventually

transforms the root cause of ingrained behaviors. No longer will pain cause us to react in ways that harm either others or ourselves. No longer will we suffer from our unconscious impulses. In this way, we will begin to heal and to gain real self-control. This does not mean that we forget or suppress the memory of a painful incident or never feel pain again. The memory is there, the pain is there; all we have changed is our unhealthy, habitual reaction to it.

Experiencing Reality

When performing breath awareness, moments of clarity and insight are occasionally experienced. Examining the mind/body phenomenon helps to understand why we do the things we do. Sitting calmly, and observing and accepting our reality as it is happening, awakens us to our true purpose—to know ourselves fully. While experiencing physical sensations and their inner movements, vibrations, and pulsations, we come to know our reality. We realize that our bodies, our thoughts, and the entire world around us are in constant flux. The more we experience changing reality, the more we can let go of attachment to it. We realize that clinging to transient feelings, sensations, thoughts, concepts, and beliefs is futile. When we are free from clinging and attachment, when we stop craving and wanting, we are liberated. It is then that we become capable of truly loving.

Just as treasures are uncovered from the earth, so virtue appears
from good deeds, and wisdom appears from a pure and peaceful mind.
To walk safely through the maze of human life, one needs the light
of wisdom and the guidance of virtue. —Attributed to Buddha

TEACHING BREATH AWARENESS TO CHILDREN

If we are to teach real peace in this world and if we are to carry on
a real war against war, we shall have to begin with the children.
—Mahatma Gandhi

You may be reading this book because you want to help your child develop more concentration or to learn how to alleviate anxiety. You may see your teenage son or daughter straying off the wholesome path, and want to offer guidance. You may be a teacher wanting a way to help your students connect with their creativity and inner selves. Whatever your motivation is for reading this book, you clearly want to help children learn how to become more empowered and happy.

Though teenagers could probably learn on their own by following the ten lessons, however, younger children benefit from the guidance of a caring and experienced adult. To help children in the best possible way, Calm Focus Joy offers two things. One, it teaches you, the adult, breath awareness. Two, it mentors you to teach children. Teaching breath awareness to children is enjoyable as it has a meaningful purpose, and is a worthwhile mission. However, teaching this particular technique comes with challenges. When you ask children to sit still and watch their breath, for example, you might encounter considerable skepticism or resistance.

Children, at least in North American society, are generally not expected to perform tasks that require focused concentration. This is not because they do not want to; nor is it because they are incapable. Simply, there are fewer opportunities that require concentration, one-pointed focus, tenacity, and skill. With each newly invented gadget, the tasks in a child's life become easier. Today's products, media, movies, and computer programs with their countless "applications" are designed for a new generation of youth who have shorter attention spans. Many of these devices have become so amazingly easy to use, that even four-year-olds can master the skills required. The idea of spending time on something seems old-fashioned; tasks that took months of focused attention and skill to accomplish in the past, can be done in nanoseconds today. With a few clicks of a mouse spelling is corrected, research completed, masterful drawings are executed, travel plans are confirmed, and a person has time remaining to social network with twenty friends before bedtime. The problem is that the more children engage in these kinds of superficial activities, the less likely their minds will grow stronger or their talents be developed.

Breath awareness, on the other hand, is not easy to do, nor is it entertaining, amusing, fun, or fast. Focusing attention on one thing for a prolonged period requires real effort, self-discipline, and time. When you first ask children if they would like to learn, you might be disheartened by their initial unenthusiastic reactions. The encouraging thing about breath awareness, however, is that once children experience its positive effects they usually want to continue. Contrary to common belief, children enjoy being calm and quiet and like to focus on their experiences, discover how their minds work, and explore their inner reality. The problem is that children are seldom encouraged to perform introspective work or given an opportunity to do so. Because breath awareness is not something children would normally try to learn by themselves, they need guidance and encouragement.

Importance of Voluntary Participation
When children practice breath awareness, adults are often surprised by their enthusiasm. Many children love doing it and intuitively know that it is a valuable skill. Their eagerness may be due to the voluntary nature of the program; only children who *choose* to learn are taught.

If a Mindmastery program is conducted in a school or community center, children usually formally apply to join. Before they commit, they must listen to an introduction that informs them about what they will be learning, in addition to the expectations and rules of the program. By completing and signing an application, they express a willingness to do the required work. Choosing to learn, without pressure from parents or peers, is crucial. As not all children are ready, it is better to wait until they are. Children who really want to learn will be motivated to perform the challenging work it takes to succeed.

The instructions in this book should be communicated gently to students without causing a feeling of pressure, restriction, or stress. The key to achieving success is to ensure that everyone who participates does so voluntarily. Even after a student has willingly joined a program, he or she may suddenly decide to quit. Again, there should never be any kind of pressure, reprimand, or persuasion to continue. If a student wishes to stop, that is his or her choice. Young people need to feel that they have control and can exercise free will. Even when a student declines to participate, he or she might still be curious and one day be interested in trying again. We never know exactly why a child might be hesitant or unwilling. There could also be underlying issues that are not obvious. Some children, for example, may really want to join but their parents or peers are cynical or make fun of what they are doing. It is best to reassure a child that it is okay not to participate.

Qualities of a Teacher
There are skills that will make you a more effective teacher. First and foremost is that you are established in practicing breath awareness. Only through actual experience of the technique's transformative power will you know how and why it works. Intellectual understanding is good, but limited. If you have practiced breath awareness for a long time, you will have gained much experiential knowledge and will know that working properly is the key to real transformation.

You can also be an effectual teacher by role modeling. Your presence and personality will inspire children more than your words. Children will sense that you are the kind of person that they can become by practicing breath awareness. They will sense your wholesome energy, peace, and wisdom—the same qualities they are aspiring to develop. They will see you taking care of your physical and mental health. If, however, your words or actions contradict the message of your teaching, students might become confused or uninspired.

To teach by example does not mean that you have to be an enlightened person, health food fanatic, or fitness instructor; it just means that you show commitment to this path. You practice daily, live in a healthy, wholesome way, and share your kindness and wisdom with others. Children will respect you more if they see that you are also a student working toward the same goals—more calmness, focus, and joy. The most important quality that will make you a wonderful teacher is compassion. If your words and actions spring from an inner source of wisdom and love, all who listen will embrace your message.

Teaching Breath Awareness
There are other important considerations to take into account when you are a teacher. Many of these are explained in the *Teacher Tips* provided in each chapter. You will learn that when it comes to doing breath awareness, more is not necessarily better. Children should not be forced to sit for long sessions; they can progress by practicing for shorter peri-

ods. A few minutes of correct technique has more value than thirty minutes of working improperly. You will also learn how to keep children working more on the surface of their minds. Although this may sound counterproductive, it is recommended that children be prevented from penetrating too deeply and too quickly into their psyche because some children suffer serious emotional and psychological problems. By working more on the surface, you ensure that trauma, anger, or overpowering sadness is not triggered. Breath awareness can release a flow of suppressed emotions that, in a classroom situation, you might simply not be equipped to deal with.

When any person, young or old, sits in one position for an extended period, it is natural to experience bodily sensations. Feet might fall asleep, the back might start aching or one may feel dizzy, light-headed, or nauseous. Although these physical sensations can be experienced by anyone at any time, if a person dwells on them while doing breath awareness, an overflow of repressed feelings may be elicited. If a student becomes overwhelmed and cannot practice breath awareness, you might offer another activity like drawing or writing. If the problem seems serious, you may want to speak with his or her parents. Sometimes, there are underlying issues that need professional help. To prevent an upsurge of negativity, your job is always to remind students to refocus on the breath. If you are not experienced, you may suddenly find yourself dealing with a child's anger, and your well-intended efforts may do more harm than good. Whenever possible, it is best to keep classes fun and humorous. Although breath awareness is a serious technique, try to make it enjoyable.

Natural Breath—Nothing More

As your students work through the ten *Student Practice Sessions*, they will learn the pure breath awareness technique, which involves being mindful of natural, normal, ordinary, unregulated, and uncontrolled respiration. The exercises require nothing more than to stay aware of the breath passing over the skin just below the entrance of the nose. It is so simple that you may want to add more. Understand, however, that adding anything to the pure technique could weaken its benefits.

Some people consider breath awareness too strict and serious for children. They feel that children, who are by nature lively and spontaneous, need exercises that allow them to express and release energy. It is true that children do need activities like dance, sports, gymnastics, and other physical ways to express themselves and to be healthy. Nevertheless, exercising attention and developing focus are also healthy activities that children enjoy. A focused mind also improves one's physical well-being.

Additionally, some people are concerned that young children will not grasp the instructions correctly. They fear that children will miscomprehend what it means to observe ordinary breathing and instead may start holding their breath or hyperventilating. It is, therefore, important to be on the lookout for this type of behavior. Some young people play the fainting game, also known as the choking game, where they intentionally cut off the brain's oxygen by holding their breath after hyperventilating to induce a euphoric feeling or hallucination. Unfortunately, this game can lead to serious brain damage and even death. Be observant of what the children are doing, as some will be curious about achieving a non-drug high while having no understanding of the consequences. Controlling the breath in any way is unadvisable and must be discouraged. If children practice breath awareness other than instructed, it is the responsibility of the teacher to educate them of the possible dangers and to stop all unsafe experimenting. Ultimately, it is up to the teacher to ensure that students practice breath awareness properly and safely. Repeatedly, the instructions in this book remind teachers and students that breath awareness requires the simple observation of natural, normal, non-regulated breathing.

A Simple Technique

Breath awareness is probably one of the simplest focus techniques available. It entails so little. You do not have to learn a variety of skills, nor do you need any special aptitude. It requires no memorization, conceptual thinking, or intellectualizing. You do not have to perform any ceremonies, rituals, chanting, or fasting. Unlike other concentration techniques, breath awareness does not employ visualization, autosuggestion, symbols, or mental images.

It is important to keep its simplicity in mind or you might be compelled to add something. For example, even though you know that no harm will come if students do slow, deep breathing, or add a word to each breath, these instructions might defeat the purpose of breath awareness. The goal is to observe *natural* breath—as it is. One moment it might be rhythmic, quiet, slow, shallow, deep, erratic, short, or long; the next moment tickly, itchy, stinging, warm, or cool. It is not possible to observe natural respiration if it is continually controlled. For this reason it is important not to mix techniques because doing so could minimize the benefits, confuse the children, and may even defeat the whole purpose of developing one's ability to observe reality. The goal is to stop controlling and imagining, and to start objectively observing one's reality—as it is.

There are countless concentration training techniques. Some of these include mindfulness, meditation, slow walking, yoga, biofeedback, visualization, insight, and sensory awareness. These techniques are certainly beneficial for training the mind and instilling calmness. Despite the multitude of benefits derived from these methods, this book teaches only *one* technique, breath awareness. Confining the instructions to one method helps students learn to practice one exercise in depth. Introducing a smorgasbord of approaches, options, and methods only confuses a beginner and dilutes the profound effects that the serious practice of breath awareness provides.

Sensory Addiction

The primary obstacle that prevents some children from focusing is their addiction to sensory stimulation. The symptoms of sensory addiction are agitation, restlessness, frustration, boredom, and hyperactive behavior. Even some very young children suffer from some form of sensory stimulation dependency. Signs of dependency include being overly impatient and fidgety, distracted, or obsessed with playing computer games or listening to iPods.

Other kinds of addictive sensory stimulation come from certain foods or substances. Some children may be mildly addicted to junk food, salt, sugar, or caffeinated soft drinks. Older children may be addicted to smoking, drugs, gambling, pornography, or alcohol. Depending on the severity of the addiction, your effort to help these children develop focus might be more difficult.

Sensory addiction is a growing trend among young people and becoming so widespread that society has come to accept it as normal. Addictions to activities like watching television usually go unnoticed. Addiction to stimulation is probably becoming a modern-day malady not yet recognized as a serious mental and physical problem by health authorities. Until sufficient data proves long-term injurious effects, there will be a tendency for the general population not to take preventative action.

Parents can control the type and amount of stimulation their children engage in. They can limit the time their children watch television or play on the computer. Even so, it is difficult to guess how little is too much. A recent study revealed that a mere nine minutes of watching a fast-paced cartoon caused short-term attention and learning problems in four year olds. There are many similar studies underway but it will be a while before there is conclusive evidence of real health risks. No one wants children to be guinea pigs in this modern-day sensory experiment. Even without facts, it seems reasonable to surmise that a child who is perpetually distracted with external stimuli will eventually suffer some kind of deficiency in their mental and physical development.

When we see children consumed by unhealthy activities, our responsibility is to minimize potential harm by calling for tactful intervention. Yet, how to intervene is not obvious. For some parents, any amount of interference in their child's fun or choices triggers rebellion and resentment.

It helps to keep up-to-date on new studies concerning the physical and mental side effects of excessive television, computer, digital and wireless device use, exposure to cell phone radioactive frequencies, along with the influences of questionable Internet sites. Children will pay attention when they are presented with facts, although sometimes reluctantly; educated debates having more weight than emotional or moral ones.

Most of us intuitively know that when computers substitute for thinking, or aid and abet memory, calculating, or problem solving, these particular mental facilities deteriorate. The old saying, *use it or lose it*, applies to brainpower just as it does to muscles.

Stimulation from entertainment may give a person a false sense of mental activity. Watching television and leisurely surfing the Internet may seem like activities where the mind is working, but unless a problem is solved, an obstacle overcome, or a goal has been achieved, minimum brainpower is generated. The activity causes more of a superficial mental buzzing, similar to the effects of caffeine, than any increase in gray matter, neural networks, or brain connectivity. Brain growth and mind development can only occur when effort is exerted to engage the mind's faculties.

Most of us, even children, suffer from at least one unhealthy habit such as a craving for or dependency on junk food, smoking, drugs, alcohol, gambling, or video games. Harmful habits and addictions of any kind can compromise health, learning, and personal growth. Television, computer games, or even social networking may not cause serious mental or physical harm like drugs or alcohol, but they do distract a child from mind-strengthening activities. If a child's formative years are spent distracted, insufficient time will remain to develop will, character, mental power, and skills.

There is no end to things that titillate the nervous system and awaken craving. We may think that shutting out external distractions is the answer; however, getting rid of all things that tempt us is impossible. And even if we did shut out the distractions, it would not solve the problem. Turning off the television or not giving your children cell phones may prevent them from becoming addicted at an early age, but unless they develop mental discipline and learn how to choose intelligently, they will always be susceptible to becoming addicted.

Stimulating and entertaining products and activities are not the actual culprits. Rather, the problem lies in our emotional and physical need to be happy, creative, and loved. We all want to feel worthwhile and to see purpose in our lives, and unless we fulfill these human desires we may remain dissatisfied, even desperate.

If playing computer games or taking drugs numbs an underlying dissatisfaction, it is natural to want to continue suppressing the pain. If communicating with friends provides a sense of belonging and purpose, it is natural to want to keep doing it. The fear of being alone drives many children and adults to depend on social networking and to seek solace in external distractions. Unfortunately, relying on external sources to alleviate the pain of loneliness may contribute to the lack of self-worth felt by many today. Without an internal focus and a strong sense of self, individuals might become susceptible to depression, hopelessness, aggression, or suicide. To prevent unwholesome mind states from consuming and controlling children, it is important that they get connected with their inner strength and wisdom. They need to experience self-confidence, power, joy, and peace in order that they do not spend their lives looking externally for fulfillment.

Understanding Today's Youth

Today's youth enjoy more time, social networking, freedom, opportunity, and entertainment than children did in the past. Today's children are free to engage in countless types of pleasure and amusement, most condoned by society and accepted as harmless pastimes. It is, however, too early to determine how social media, entertainment, television, telephones, and computers are shaping the minds of our children.

What we do know is that overexposure to stimulation in a child's formative years conditions thinking and behavior. Once conditioning becomes ingrained it is difficult to change and could have serious effects causing a person to become indifferent, aggressive, antisocial, racist, or to assume a distorted view of sexuality.

Strengthening the mind takes time and effort. When seductive, endorphin-stimulating entertainment lures children away from activities that require stamina and effort, like learning a skill or concentrating on one thing, there remains little time for mind development. When time is spent on entertainment, children cannot enhance their mental faculties like intellect, memory, perception, cognition, and attention. Overstimulation may diminish natural curiosity and cause boredom, apathy, or depression. The distressing thing is that children can also develop these unenthusiastic mind states and emotions and, if they have never experienced otherwise, they will not know what they are missing.

Children might also not see the point of breath awareness as the rewards are neither immediate nor visible. Children thrive on instant gratification and generally have not been instilled with the old-fashioned work ethic, *sow now, reap later*. A century ago, young people understood this ethic because the circumstances of life did not give them many other options. You worked now for what you received later; you learned skills while young so you could survive in adulthood. There were few frivolous distractions from learning or working and delaying gratification was a sign of maturity and vision. Children spent their early years working, building, farming, hunting, raising siblings, or learning a trade. Privileged children born into affluence may have enjoyed more leisure time, but nothing quite like it is today.

Today, in technologically advanced and wealthy societies, working for survival is not foremost on a young person's mind and there is ample time for pleasure and entertainment. We cannot hold it against children for choosing titillating distractions over laborious skill-developing work. After all, it is instinctive to choose the path of least resistance.

Awakening Curiosity

Once you realize that children will benefit by improving their focus and gaining self-knowledge, how do you convince them to do the work?

How you get them to willingly sign up for a Mindmastery program or similar courses that practice mind-strengthening exercises? With hundreds of distractions competing for attention, how do you inspire a young person to learn breath awareness? Perhaps there is little we can say or do to convince a child to develop concentration. Fortunately, the problem of convincing solves itself when children start doing breath awareness. After one session, many experience more calmness and energy, and as a result feel motivated to continue. After only a few sessions of breath awareness, students usually experience noticeable changes and feel more confident and relaxed.

As breath awareness starts to cause inner transformation, many children, even as young as eight years old, show growing social awareness and compassion. They write in their journals about making the world a more peaceful place, protecting animals and the environment, and even wanting to stop racism and wars. As they become more considerate and respectful toward their friends, teachers, and parents, their kind thoughts and actions inspire respect and appreciation. When a child is valued in this manner, he or she feels happy. Every person wants to feel worthwhile and appreciated. When these emotional needs are fulfilled, a person relies less on superficial, short-lived stimulation, or cyberspace friendships for happiness and self-worth.

Parents and teachers are primarily responsible for children's education and upbringing. Would it not be wise to teach skills to children that nurture confidence and well-being? Of all the subjects taught in school and at home, should focus training, introspection, and awakening self-awareness not rank top on the list? Helping children learn these important lessons is the most valuable kind of education we can offer. If children can master their restless minds enough to reflect on who they are, they will do better in all areas of their lives.

Children who experience breath awareness acquire the technique for life. Similar to riding a bicycle, even if you do not continue, you will never forget how to do it. Once calmness, confidence, and focus have been experienced, the memory of breath awareness becomes a dormant seed planted in the mind. When a child grows older and faces difficult decisions or emotional turbulence, he or she will remember what to do. Although you might not be there to witness this moment you can be confident that the seed you planted will be there. A child will always remember the power of breath. Children who learn breath awareness and continue to practice throughout their lives learn more about who they are, self-knowledge being the best protection against the onslaught of harmful, misleading external influences in a world that can be daunting. A person who is strong within has the courage and confidence to confront all of life's challenges.

Many of us feel inadequate or powerless when it comes to rectifying the conditions of the world. Nevertheless, we possess the power to change ourselves. Personal transformation is the first step toward making a difference in the world. We may think that developing ourselves will have little impact. However, all we have to do is think about any one of the thousands of individuals who have had a positive effect on this planet. They are the wise men, saints, artists, philosophers, writers, musicians, scientists, doctors, visionaries, and teachers who all made a difference. These men and women were inwardly developed, inspired, focused, intelligent, and motivated to make a change. They shared a reverence for life and compassion for human suffering. By establishing strength, peace, and benevolence within themselves, they inspired millions of people to follow their own inner paths.

If each of us establishes harmony within, our external world will become one of peace and tolerance. If we master our minds and govern our bodies we will transform humanity. It is for this reason that cultivating the minds of our children is essential. The state of tomorrow's world depends on the state of our children's minds today. None of these changes can happen through the use of force because, like anyone, children must discover their own life purpose as an individual pursuit. They alone can find an internal focus that sparks and sustains their interest.

What we can do is provide children with guidance, opportunity, and encouragement to investigate who they are. This kind of introspective education will pave the way to helping children discover their purpose. The more connected they become with their inner truth, the more they will know themselves. When they know who they are and how they want to be, they will choose their path with confidence. There are many ways to encourage children to reconnect with their inner selves. Our job is to help. Teaching breath awareness is one of many beneficial lessons. By encouraging children to spend time learning about themselves we are sending a message. We are saying that their mental, emotional, and spiritual well-being is of the utmost importance.

Selfless Sharing

Breath awareness develops compassion and selflessness. Your students will be inspired when they see these qualities in you. They will be touched to know that you are giving them a gift without expecting anything in return. Giving selflessly benefits both you and your students.

Mindmastery programs or breath awareness lessons should be offered free of any charge. Even asking for donations could compromise the power of pure selfless giving. If you are in a life situation that does not allow you to give the time or some expense to facilitate a program, it is best to wait until your circumstances change.

Teaching breath awareness without charging a fee allows everyone—rich or poor, young or old, weak or strong, healthy or handicapped—to feel good about participating. Receiving something free is rare in today's world, so when a person receives a selfless gift, it can have an amazing impact. Selflessness and generosity motivate others to share in the same way. You might find that people who have benefited from what they have learned will want to help financially, by donating materials, or volunteering their time. Accepting charity in order to continue your selfless giving may be something that happens while walking this path. Your volition will be pure and whatever gifts you graciously receive will ultimately benefit others.

Keep the Technique Pure

When teaching breath awareness to children or facilitating the Mindmastery Program, it is recommended that the lessons be delivered exactly as instructed. Try not to mix, change, or add anything. As well, when learning the technique on your own, follow *Your Practice* instructions as closely as you can. Observe how pure breath awareness works for you. If you notice a change in your disposition, if your concentration improves, if you gain insight into your mind/body phenomenon, or if you feel more inspired to help others, you will know that breath awareness is working.

MINDMASTERY PROGRAM OVERVIEW

Mindmastery or the *Mindmastery Program* is the name given to the ten breath awareness lessons presented in this book. Mindmastery is a word easily understood by children, teenagers, and adults and clearly describes the primary goal of breath awareness. Children, whether they are five or fifteen, especially like the idea of gaining mastery over their restless and distracted minds. Being young and with limited choice, young people embrace the prospect of governing their lives. They also understand, at least intuitively, the benefits of becoming more focused, confident, and self-disciplined.

The ten-step Mindmastery Program presents a holistic method that incorporates three fundamental ingredients that human beings need to be happy: *autonomy*—making one's own choices; *mastery*—acquiring and performing a skill well; and *purpose*—doing something for the well-being of others.

Breath awareness is a technique used to calm the mind and develop focus. However, practicing breath awareness alone would not give the best results. To achieve long-lasting transformation, the technique incorporates three other important components: *wholesome conduct*—living without harming others or oneself; *awakening insight*—developing self-knowledge and wisdom; and *sharing goodwill*—sharing thoughts of love, kindness, peace and happiness with others. When a person practices these aspects along with breath awareness, he or she will progress steadily and realize significant positive changes.

The book offers three levels of instruction. The first, called *Your Practice* teaches breath awareness to adults in ten progressive steps The second level of instruction is found in *Student Instructions* and *Student Practice Sessions*. These lessons can be read aloud or rephrased more simply to teach breath awareness to a single child or a group of chil dren. The third level of instruction is found under the headings *Teacher Tips, Facilitating a Mindmastery Program,* and *You, the Teacher*. These sections provide in-depth explanations on the theory and practice of breath awareness and offer ways to explain it to children using anecdotes and stories. These sections also offer suggestions on organizing and conducting your own breath awareness program.

When you read through the chapters, you will notice significant repetition. Keep in mind that you are reading three different levels of instruction that all teach the same technique. Although the information may seem redundant, you will gain a thorough intellectual understanding of the technique's theory and practice.

Before you teach breath awareness to others, work through all ten *Your Practice* sessions. To do this, simply read *Your Practice* instructions, perform the practical exercise, and then, if you wish, reflect on the questions found in *Check-in*. To further deepen your experience and integrate what you are learning into daily life, you may try the suggestions offered in the *Continuation of Practice Tip.*

While working through each step, you may also enjoy reading *Teacher Tips*. These provide in-depth explanations of the technique aimed to help you progress in your own practice and, as well, help you teach children. *Student Instructions* and *Student Practice Sessions* present read-aloud breath awareness instructions written specifically for a younger audience.

Become the Light

If your goal is to teach your child, children, or students, there is no question that your first step is to become firmly established in breath awareness. They say that Buddha's final words before he passed away were, "Be a light unto thy self." These words sum up the true path to becoming an influential teacher. First, become a light; then will you be a North Star for others.

It is not necessary to read the whole book before you begin the practical work. In fact, it may be more productive to progress through lessons one step at a time. The ten sessions can comfortably be completed in about two weeks, but could be condensed or lengthened to suit your time schedule. Condensing several steps into a few days could be beneficial. An intense program would require that you practice several hours per day, which would give you an insightful and transformative experience.

Alternatively, if you are just beginning to learn breath awareness, it might be best to work through one lesson each day. This pace would allow you to incorporate breath awareness into your daily routine. Others may prefer stretching the ten lessons out over a few months by completing one step each week. This approach would also work, provided you continue to practice regularly. Whichever way you decide to proceed, positive transformation happens when you practice every day.

Although practicing daily is the most challenging aspect of doing breath awareness, it is the secret to success.

Even if teaching children is not your ambition, once you start enjoying the benefits of your practice you might change your mind. As often happens after experiencing more inner peace, one naturally feels like sharing the technique with others.

Selfless giving just happens and is a by-product of practicing breath awareness. When this transpires, you may want to introduce breath awareness to your children, partner, students, friends, or patients. Working through the chapters and learning breath awareness on your own will give you the experience to know what to expect, how to overcome obstacles, and how to heal negative mind states. Your experience will give you knowledge that will make it easier to explain breath awareness to others.

Ideally, you will not have to rely on the book when you teach, but rather you will impart your wisdom in your own words. Children usually enjoy listening without the intervention of a book. If teaching is your goal, you may eventually want to conduct a program in your home, school, or community. This book provides extensive information on how to organize and facilitate a full Mindmastery program or how to teach breath awareness in a lesson or two. Information for future teachers can be found under the headings *Teacher Tips, You, the Teacher, Facilitating a Mindmastery Program, Sample Application Form, Student and Teacher Experience*, and *Questions and Answers*.

Student Introduction Part I and Part II
It is crucial to deliver the two-part student introduction to children who are interested in attending a Mindmastery program or in learning breath awareness. Anyone who wants to join must be well informed about course expectations, and be clear about what they will be doing and the benefits to be gained. It is imperative that students listen to Part I and Part II *before* agreeing to join a program.

With this requirement, each student can make an informed decision whether or not to participate. Informed students who join because they like what they hear and are up for the challenge will have the incentive to work seriously, follow the rules, persevere, and be successful. Since parents play an essential role in their children's education, they are always welcome to attend student introduction sessions where they can ask questions and become familiar with what their children will be learning. Their encouragement and support will further motivate their children to work harder and to feel good about practicing at home.

The Ten-Step Mindmastery Program

The Mindmastery Program comprises ten learning steps for both adults and children. The program concludes with two post-steps. Each lesson starts with an explanation of the technique followed by practical instructions. Each step includes eight components:

1. *Your Practice*: A personal coaching session for the adult learner.
2. *Teacher Tips*: Explanations and advice on how to teach children.
3. *Student Instructions*: Read-aloud instructions for children.
4. *Student Practice Session*: A guided breath awareness session for children of all ages.
5. *Story*: A humorous tale illustrating breath awareness theory and practice for young children.
6. *Student Journal*: Writing and art suggestions.
7. *Check-in*: Questions to help the adult monitor progress and reflect on experience following a breath awareness session.
8. *Continuation of Practice Tip:* Suggestions on incorporating breath awareness in daily life.

1) Your Practice

At the beginning of each step, you will find a section called *Your Practice*. These guidelines provide adult learners with a personalized instruction guide. To learn breath awareness, proceed through each of the ten *Your Practice* sessions. While doing these sessions you may also enjoy reading *Teacher Tips*, which provide further insight into the technique.

2) Teacher Tips

This section follows *Your Practice*. It provides in-depth explanations of breath awareness and its theory. The information enriches an adult's understanding of how breath awareness works and prepares him or her for teaching the upcoming student lesson.

3) Student Instructions

These instructions are written in a read-aloud format so they can be read directly out of the book. Although it would be better for a teacher to deliver the instructions and explanations in his or her own words,

Student Instructions provide a clear guideline for giving breath awareness instructions to a group of children. Before students perform each practical exercise, these instructions explain how the technique works in easy-to-understand language.

4) Student Practice Session

These instructions are also written in a script-like format so they can be read aloud to students. Giving prompts while students are doing breath awareness is intuitive and a teacher should only say something when necessary. After listening to the explanations, instructions, and theory, students perform a practical breath awareness exercise. A teacher may paraphrase or edit these read-aloud instructions, delivering them in whatever words work best for the level of his or her pupils. *Student Practice Sessions* get progressively longer. However, the teacher will ultimately decide how long breath awareness sessions should be. For restless, young, or hyperactive children, the suggested sitting times can be adjusted to a few minutes.

5) Stories

Every step concludes with a fun children's story or fairy tale, which illustrates how breath awareness can be used in life. These stories are meant for young children, but could be revised to suit older students.

6) Student Journal

At the end of each *Student Practice Session* students are encouraged to write or draw in a journal, which helps them intellectually process what they are experiencing. After sitting still and experiencing new things about themselves children feel creative and expressive. Accommodating their urge to write, paint, draw, or talk is important. All forms of expression are encouraged. If some children prefer not to write or do anything, that is fine. As long as they are not disruptive, they can sit, relax, and observe. In the chapter *Student and Teacher Experience* you will find insightful excerpts from past students' journals.

7) Check-in

Check-in questions help you reflect on your breath awareness experiences. They help clarify and deepen understanding, keep you on track, eliminate confusion, and indicate your progress. You may use some of the *Check-in* questions for younger students, but not all are relevant to what they are learning.

8) Continuation of Practice Tip

Concluding each chapter is a *Continuation of Practice Tip* suggesting a way to deepen your practice and to incorporate breath awareness into daily life.

The Importance of Step Ten - Sharing Goodwill

Sharing Goodwill is an additional technique that students perform after they have practiced breath awareness and are feeling peaceful. This ancient technique is also known as loving-kindness meditation or Metta. By Step Ten, most students will feel more peaceful and compassionate toward other living beings and even themselves. When they feel kindness and joy, they are ready for this final lesson.

Sharing is an important aspect of breath awareness. Sending out thoughts of goodwill cultivates selflessness and promotes happiness. Children who practice sharing their peace and harmony begin to understand that what they are doing and the demanding work they are performing is not just to benefit themselves but others as well. They begin to realize that they can generate healing energy and can send this energy to help their friends, family, and community.

Post-steps

Breath Awareness for Life and *Healthy Body–Healthy Mind* are the two post-steps that conclude the Mindmastery Program. They provide suggestions on how to continue practicing breath awareness at home while emphasizing the maintenance of a healthy lifestyle.

You, the Teacher

Suggestions and recommendations prepare you to teach children breath awareness and to facilitate a Mindmastery program.

Facilitating a Mindmastery Program

Invaluable and detailed information provide guidelines on how to organize and teach breath awareness to a group of children in your home, school, or community.

Sample Application Form

If you are planning to conduct a ten-step Mindmastery program or just teach a few sessions of breath awareness in a school, club, camp, or community center, you might require application forms, letters to parents, and other written material. In this chapter you will find sample applications and letters that can be revised to suit your needs.

Requesting that children apply to attend a program serves several purposes. First, formally applying to Mindmastery ensures that a child is joining willingly and that he or she has read the rules of the program and has agreed to follow them. Second, application forms provide a way to collect important information including parent or guardian contact numbers, doctor's name, allergies or health issues, special needs, or psychological concerns. The forms also request that parents and guardians give their consent along with signing a waiver releasing all persons of liability. Please note that the liability release offered in this book is a guideline and should not be used without being examined and rewritten by a professional. By doing your due diligence, you will be guaranteed coverage in case of an accident, emergency, or lawsuit.

Questions and Answers
Answers to frequently asked questions help clear up confusion about breath awareness. Even though the technique is straightforward, many students have legitimate concerns. The explanations provided in this chapter should help students understand intellectually what they are doing and help them feel confident about the technique so they can work properly and benefit from their efforts.

Student and Teacher Experience
A selection of journal excerpts written by children and adults communicate insightful observations about their experiences.

Research
Neuroscientific research is finding that breath awareness and other mindfulness and meditation techniques can significantly help brain functions, reduce stress, and improve health. This chapter presents excerpts from several current studies in this field.

STUDENT INTRODUCTION - PART I

Joining a Mindmastery Program

The following two-part student introduction provides read-aloud information for children who are interested in participating in a Mindmastery program. These talks explain the essential aspects of breath awareness, the benefits that come from developing focus, the role of wholesome conduct, and how mastering the restless mind can increase one's happiness, health, and empathy for others. Before children agree to learn breath awareness, they should understand program expectations, what they will be doing, and what results they can expect to achieve.

Read-Aloud Introduction

Thank you for your interest in the Mindmastery Program. Mindmastery is a challenging, yet fun course that teaches you how to do *breath awareness*. Breath awareness is a simple exercise that can help to improve focus, calm restlessness, and awaken insights into how your mind works. The primary aim of doing breath awareness is to strengthen your attention "muscle". Through developing strong and sharp attention skills, you will be able to think more clearly, understand complex subjects, learn faster, and have the capability to achieve goals. If you can focus, you will do well in all areas of your life including school, sports, work, and friendships. If you are peaceful and calm, you will feel empowered, confident, and happy about yourself.

Practicing breath awareness helps to develop the brain and its faculties. The exercise of focusing improves attention, intellect, memory, perception, cognition, comprehension, imagination, and intuition. It also helps to develop mindmastery, self-discipline, and wisdom. When you master your distracted mind and curb unwholesome habits, you will be capable of achieving amazing things in your life.

Breath awareness requires that you examine only one thing, that is, your breath. When you focus on one thing, you usually awaken interest and curiosity, which leads to greater understanding about the thing you are studying. Whenever you become keenly interested in something, learning becomes meaningful and enjoyable.

In this technique, you will learn everything there is to know about your breath. You will discover how your breath directly influences your state of mind. You will learn how breath connects you with your thoughts, sensations, feelings, aspirations, and even the unconscious part of your mind. You will learn how your thoughts can influence feelings, and how your feelings can influence your thinking. All the knowledge that you gain will come from your own experiences, not through reading books or listening to lectures.

When you participate in Mindmastery, you will be taught how to practice breath awareness properly. This will require that you sit silently, pay attention to your breathing, and feel the touch of your incoming and outgoing breath near the entrance of your nose. You will begin practicing for five or ten minutes and gradually work up to longer periods. The exercise may sound easy, but doing breath awareness takes sustained effort, which is not easy. Even grown ups have difficulty keeping their attentions focused on one thing for more than a few minutes.

When you try to focus only on breathing, your mind naturally gets restless. Your attention hates being focused and would rather jump from one interesting thought to the next. Jumping around has become its habit. Your inability to attend to one thing at a time is a sign that your attention muscle is weak. A weak and scattered attention will not help you become a more happy, healthy, and peaceful person. As well, a person whose mind is continually distracted and agitated will not be able to contribute to the peace and harmony of our world. Therefore, if you want to make a difference in your own life or you wish to help the world become a better place, the first step is to develop and strengthen your mind.

As you work through the Mindmastery sessions, you will begin to recognize different sensations, feelings, and emotions. One day you may feel agitated, frustrated, restless, bored, unhappy, or angry. The next, you may feel elated, excited, happy, or calm. You will learn how to objectively observe these different emotions, aches, and pains without reacting to them.

Developing the ability to objectively observe what is happening inside of your mind and body is a valuable skill. For example, when you are frustrated with homework you might start texting your friends or going on Facebook. Unfortunately, time passes quickly when you are distracted and you might not complete your homework. This could result in bad grades or failing a test. Learning to recognize frustration before reacting to it, gives you a choice. You can choose to ignore the frustration and get on with your homework or you can choose not to text your friends. Both of these choices will help you develop more focus, self-discipline, and achieve good grades.

Breath awareness also awakens compassion and caring for others. When you hear about children starving or dying of disease in another country, you will feel empathetic. You may then want to help and initiate a fundraiser for food and medical supplies. Your generosity and kindness will inspire others to do similar work or to help you with your mission.

Before agreeing to join Mindmastery, it is a good idea to learn a little more about what you will be doing. The main activity will be breath awareness. Before each practice session, the instructor will explain a few things about the technique. Then, when you start sitting, you will be guided along. There should be no need to worry whether or not you can do this exercise. Whenever you have a question, just ask. After each sitting, there will be time for writing and art.

There are four parts, or aspects, to learning breath awareness. When you work through the program, you will be taught all four to ensure long-lasting, positive benefits. The first fundamental component of breath awareness is *wholesome conduct*. Wholesome conduct means to live, act, speak, or behave in a way that does not harm anyone, including yourself. This includes behaviors like unhealthy habits and addictions. Unwholesome and habitual behaviors are those things we do without thinking or having control over. Making wholesome, healthy choices, and refraining from hurting others prevents your mind from becoming severely agitated. If your mind is relatively calm and peaceful before you begin practicing breath awareness, focusing will be easier and you will progress faster.

The second component is *breath awareness*—the focus training technique used to strengthen the attention and calm the mind. Breath awareness requires one to sit quietly, be mindful of the incoming and outgoing breath, and make an effort not to react to feelings of restlessness, agitation, or boredom.

The third component of this technique usually happens on its own after you have been practicing for a while. This aspect is known as *awakening insight.* Awakening insight describes those flashes of understanding and wisdom that naturally occur when you are investigating your mind and body sensations. The more connected you become with sensations felt by the breath, the more you understand how sensations, feelings, and thoughts are constantly changing. These insights help you know to yourself more deeply.

The fourth component also happens naturally when you practice seriously. It is called *sharing goodwill.* Sharing goodwill means exactly that—to share your positive energy and happiness with others. You will learn how to send out thoughts of loving kindness to help your family, friends, pets, community, and even strangers. After several sessions of breath awareness, you usually start to feel more peaceful and happy. When this happens, you will be ready to share goodwill.

It may be helpful to explain what you will actually be doing when you practice breath awareness. First, you will be instructed to sit still and not speak for five to ten minutes and focus your attention on your breath. As you develop greater ability to concentrate you will be able do breath awareness for longer stretches. After ten sessions, some students find sitting forty-five minutes relatively easy. In the beginning, however, sitting for a few minutes is a great achievement.

You will be sitting cross-legged or in a kneeling position on a cushion on the floor. If this is uncomfortable, sitting on the edge of a chair is an option. Whichever sitting position you choose, your back will be straight, your hands will be folded in your lap or resting on your knees, and for most of the session, your eyes will be closed.

Once you are quiet and comfortable, you will then be instructed to fix your attention on your breath and feel it touch the small area of skin in and around your nostrils. For the whole time, your attention will focus on feeling the breath's delicate, warm touch passing over the small area of skin below your nose and above your upper lip. Breath awareness requires you to stop thinking and to start feeling.

The first thing that you may discover when you try breath awareness is that your thoughts keep jumping around. One minute you may be thinking about a past event; the next minute you may be imagining the future. Getting distracted is normal for the untrained mind. Ever since we were born, our attention has been busily jumping from one thought to the next. This jumping around has become our mind's biggest habit. As you know, habits are hard to change. The moment we choose to train our attention and keep it focused on one thing, we start to change this habit. The more we change this habit, the more mastery we develop. Being the master of your mind gives you power and control, making you the boss and decision-maker of who you want to be, what you want to do, and how you want to live.

How about we try doing breath awareness for a minute or two? Sit up straight. Tuck in your chin. Fold your hands in your lap and close your eyes. Now, breathe in. Can you feel your breath? Is it warm or is it cool? Now, breathe out. Can you feel your breath inside your nose or touching just below your nostrils? What temperature is it? Breathing in and breathing out with awareness is simple to do but, as you can see, requires real effort. Doing it for five minutes sounds insignificant, but is actually a great start. Well done. You can now open your eyes. How was it? Could you feel the touch of breath? Did your mind jump around? Were you able to stay focused on your breath?

Attending a Mindmastery program will be challenging, however, it may be the best thing you ever do for yourself. Here is a story that illustrates the importance of developing mastery over the restless, out-of-control mind.

Wild Elephants of the Jungle

Once upon a time, deep in the jungles of India, there lived a tribe of peaceful and hardworking farmers. For many years, the tribe was plagued by a terrible problem—the wild elephants of the jungle. Every year, just before harvest time, the terrifying elephants would charge toward their village with a thundering rumble and trumpeting cries. Fearing for their lives, men and women would grab their children and scramble up the tallest trees.

From there, they would watch in horror while hundreds of out-of-control beasts trampled their huts, broke their fences, and destroyed their fields. When the dust settled, the elephants were gone and the heartbroken villagers would climb down the trees to survey the damage. Every time, they would see the same discouraging devastation. Year after year, the wild elephants would return and ruin everything. Feeling powerless and perplexed, the wise chief and all the elders believed that their tribe had been cursed forever.

Now, after overhearing the elders discuss the reoccurring disaster, a young boy pondered the problem for several days. Early one morning, when no one was paying attention, he secretly ran away into the jungle. He walked alone for two whole days. Finally, he found what he was looking for. Far below, in a lush valley, he spied the terrifying elephant herd grazing with their young. The boy waited until midnight. When the elephants were asleep, he quietly snuck down between them and found a baby elephant sleeping. He made a soft sound to wake it up. Then he used a peanut to coax it to come closer to him. The little elephant was curious and shyly walked toward the boy. As soon as it was near, the boy slipped a rope around its head and led it away.

Back at the village, the tribe had been searching for the boy for days. Days turned to months. Finally, believing that he had been killed in the stampede, they sadly gave up their search.

A year went by, and it was harvest time. The villagers prepared themselves for the terrible day when the elephants would charge through their village. The day came sooner than expected. They heard a distant shrill of a trumpet— the battle cry of elephants. Men, women, and children scrambled up the trees to safety and watched in terror.

However, instead of charging elephants, out from the jungle came a boy riding a small elephant. The elephant was pulling a cart filled with rocks and logs. The boy looked up to everyone and cried, "My people, fear no more! We are not a cursed tribe, but a blessed one. We no longer need to fear the wild elephants. Look, how strong and gentle my baby elephant has become. What we must do is tame and train the wild elephants of the jungle. Let them work for us!"

From that day on, they trained the elephants to work for them and the elephants soon became the tribe's greatest asset. They used the elephants to help with logging, building, and cultivating their fields. With the elephants' help, their crops increased. They had so much food they shared it with neighboring tribes. Whenever the boy had time, he rode his elephant friend great distances and helped others learn how to train the wild elephants of the jungle.

It is probably clear that the story of the wild elephants illustrates how we can train our out-of-control minds to work for us instead of against us. Your mind is more powerful than an elephant, but you must learn to harness that power if you want to be happy and successful in life.

You have now learned more about the Mindmastery Program and the breath awareness technique. If you are interested in joining the upcoming program, please stay and listen to the second part of this introduction, which explains more thoroughly the importance of wholesome conduct. Thank your for interest and we look forward to working together to help you achieve more focus and calmness.

STUDENT INTRODUCTION - PART II

Importance of Wholesome Conduct

When we embark on the journey to strengthen our minds and to establish peace within, most of us would agree that it should not be a superficial or temporary experience. As well, after working diligently to develop focus, we would not want to compromise our goal of becoming more peaceful and happy. The effort we undertake and the hours we spend sharpening our minds should pay off in a good way. To ensure that your hard work will not be in vain you must begin your journey with a solid foundation. Like an anchor, establishing a firm internal foundation will keep you from drifting off course and ending up somewhere less than ideal. The way to develop inner fortitude and moral integrity is to conduct yourself in a wholesome manner. This means to do or say things that are healthy and life affirming while avoiding behaviors that harm you or others. To succeed at achieving your goals, it helps to develop *wholesome conduct.*

Wholesome is defined as good, kind, beneficial, caring, healthy, empathetic, natural, decent, ethical, moral, selfless, generous, uplifting, and compassionate. *Conduct* implies behavior, action, speech, thought, and intention, and encompasses how we speak to people, do business, deal with relationships, treat others, make a living, and care for our health and the welfare of others. Together, the words *wholesome conduct* mean that what you do or say promotes happiness, health, kindness, and well-being.

Wholesome conduct is essential if a person wants to cultivate the kind of focus that leads to more happiness, health, and wisdom. Performing unwholesome actions ultimately agitates the mind making it extremely difficult to develop focus and to achieve such goals. If your mind remains overly disturbed, you will be unable to establish the inner stillness needed for breath awareness and introspective investigation.

When you harm someone or yourself with harsh thoughts, words or actions, your mind gets agitated. It is agitated not because someone told it to be, but rather because agitation is a natural consequence of unwholesome behavior. Even when you do not openly express your anger or frustration, agitation will brew for some time making your mind restless. If feelings escalate, it becomes increasingly difficult to contain them. Without even knowing why, you may lose control and lash out at someone, or even yourself. Even after you lash out, agitation does not stop. After an emotional outburst, the uncomfortable restlessness, depression, worry, remorse, guilt, or unhappiness perpetuate and you remain trapped in the cycle of agitation.

You now understand more clearly how wholesome conduct supports breath awareness and helps you develop more mindmastery. Therefore, while working through this program, it is recommended that you refrain from behavior that will agitate your mind. Here are seven wholesome conduct promises that will help to build a solid foundation so you can progress steadily toward your goals.

Seven Wholesome Conduct Promises

1) I promise to respect life and not to kill any living creature.
2) I promise to respect the property of others and not steal.
3) I promise to speak truthfully and to act honestly.
4) I promise to refrain from sexual misconduct.
5) I promise to not take drugs or intoxicants.
6) I promise to refrain from hurtful speech.
7) I promise to not hurt or harm anyone or myself.

1) I Promise to Respect Life and to Not Kill any Living Creature
This seems like an easy promise to keep, as you could not imagine killing anyone. However, when we promise to respect life, this includes *all* life and living creatures. Even when we kill an animal or an insect we are not respecting life as much as we could, and these actions cause our minds to become agitated. We might not notice it at first, but once we try to do breath awareness it will be difficult to focus.

Questions concerning justifiable killing are difficult to answer. We know that we do not *want* to kill, but what if we are asked to defend our country, protect our family, or accept the death penalty? How do we answer when the issue concerns compassionate killing or assisting the death of a person who is in a coma? What do we do when someone is drowning and we know we would also drown if we tried to help? How do we survive without killing animals for food?

When you practice breath awareness you develop wisdom and compassion. When your mind is free from negative states such as selfishness, anger, racism, hate, or fear and when you have gained mastery over your blind reactions, you will be able to answer these questions more easily. If you eat meat, you might choose an alternative protein. If you must defend your country, you might ask for a position or duty that does not require killing. If you are forced to take another person's life in self-defense or because it saves an innocent person, you will do this act with more compassion.

Another activity that many of us do, without even thinking how it can agitate the mind, is *virtual* killing. Humans are often attracted to things whereby they can vicariously experience death, destruction, fear, danger, morbidity, and horror. Many children, teenagers, and adults enjoy or even become addicted to the intoxicating sensation of playing aggressive video games or watching violent movies. Even though actual life is not destroyed, the fantasy of killing and the morbidity of death can be enthralling—perhaps similar to taking drugs or doing something violent or aggressive. Virtual killing, in any form, agitates the mind and makes concentrating on the breath more difficult.

2) I Promise to Respect the Property of Others and to Not Steal
This seems like an easy promise to keep; none of us wants to steal. However, even taking something seemingly insignificant without asking, such as someone's crayon, candy, or hairbrush, can cause harm. When your mind becomes agitated you take something that does not belong to you, you make another person unhappy. Even if you justify stealing, no amount of denial will stop your mind from becoming restless, guilt-ridden, or remorseful.

3) I Promise to Speak Truthfully and to Act Honestly
None of us wants to lie, deceive, con, swindle, mislead, misinform, manipulate, or betray another person. Sometimes, however, it is very difficult to keep this promise to act completely honestly; for example, when our parents ask us what we did after school, we might mention the acceptable things but not disclose the full truth. If we create untrue stories about someone else or ourselves, we are also being dishonest. If we cheat in a game, on a test, or in a relationship, these actions cause our minds to become disturbed. It takes courage to be honest and to tell the

truth. Most of us fear the consequences of our deceit; we do not want to reveal our weakness or fear. We want our parents to be proud of us, our partners to love us, and our peers to respect us. Nevertheless, the pain of telling the truth is temporary; the trust you cultivate when you are honest and apologize if necessary, lasts a lifetime.

4) I Promise to Refrain from Sexual Misconduct

Sex is a natural activity, bonding two people in a loving relationship. It is integral to family life and the survival of our race. It can be a beautiful expression of feelings and can promote health and well-being. Sex is not something to be avoided. However, becoming obsessed or addicted to sexual stimulation can make it an unhealthy, unwholesome activity. Addiction of any kind compromises one's personal freedom, health, and happiness. Addiction to sexual stimulation can cause the mind to become very agitated, making breath awareness difficult.

With the Internet, magazines, books, television, video games, and movies we have easy access to infinite sexual images. Some of these pictures or movies are aggressive, degrading, offensive, or abusive. Even if you realize that the people in these films or photographs are only actors, the images might cause sensations that might lead to craving, which ultimately causes the mind to become agitated. Sexual images evoke pleasurable sensations and it is easy to develop an obsession or addiction toward them. However, any addiction or obsession for particular sensations compromises self-control and causes the mind to be restless, frustrated, excited, or agitated. Performing breath awareness and achieving mental calm and one-pointed focus will be difficult as a result.

5) I Promise to Not Take Drugs or Other Intoxicants

This is a difficult promise to keep because our society condones certain drugs and intoxicants. The problem is that alcohol and drugs can dull or damage the mind. A dull mind cannot develop sharp focus or observe objectively, which are skills needed when doing breath awareness. If we cannot focus, we cannot cultivate happiness and health, or achieve our goals. Even moderate drinking or drug use can lead to addiction. An addiction takes away our freedom and causes mental and emotional problems. If you presently suffer an addiction, breath awareness will be more challenging.

To ensure success, try to abstain from drugs and alcohol while working through the Mindmastery Program. There is a good chance that you will find quitting your habit easier after practicing breath awareness and gaining more control over your habit-mind. Make a strong determination to refrain from taking drugs, consuming alcohol, or smoking. Remember, any substance that excites, dulls, induces hallucinations, weakens, or pacifies the mind will make breath awareness more difficult. Your mind is your most valuable asset; keeping it healthy rewards you with more focus and happiness.

6) I Promise to Refrain from Hurtful Speech

This is the most difficult promise to keep because speaking negatively of others is something we all do without thinking twice. It is common to put others down in order to make ourselves feel superior. The sensation of superiority can be addictive. If we boast, *Look how much more popular I am than those other kids,* <u>we</u> end up feeling miserable. Our words hurt both the person we are speaking about and disturb our own peace.

There are times when it is essential to examine critically what people say or do. It is also courageous to speak our opinions and to expose corruption. The key is to ensure that our minds are pure before we voice our opinions. In this way, our criticism will be objective, well meaning, and constructive. Before putting others down, examine your intention and state of mind. If you are criticizing just to make yourself feel better or to devastate others, refrain from speaking until you can rephrase your comments.

7) I Promise to Not Hurt or Harm Others or Myself

Some people bully and insult others by calling them names, spreading lies on the Internet, or committing aggressive acts that cause harm. The reason for learning breath awareness is to become aware of the conditioning that causes us to do hurtful things. Only if we transform ourselves at the deepest levels can we change.

By keeping these seven wholesome conduct promises, especially while learning breath awareness, you will progress steadily and enjoy more focus. You will also be become the kind of people that others trust, love, and can count on.

About "Your Practice"

Your Practice sessions, found at the beginning of every step, offer personalized instructions that teach the adult or older teen the breath awareness technique in a systematic and progressive way. There are ten lessons, each requiring about one hour for reading the instructions and performing the practical work. Each lesson sets out guidelines for your sitting session and becomes progressively more challenging to ensure that you experience profound transformation.

Along with *Your Practice*, you will find another helpful section called *Check-in*. Here several reflective questions are asked to help keep you on track and to check your progress. Concluding *Check-in* you will find a *Continuation of Practice Tip*, which suggests ways to incorporate what you have learned into your daily life.

While working through *Your Practice* sessions, you may enjoy reading other sections in the book. However, keep in mind that it is not necessary to read the whole book before you begin. It is better to proceed through the book one step at a time. By being methodical, you will gain experiential knowledge that will help you grasp the technique's theory.

Establish a Daily Routine

You will find it beneficial to establish a daily routine. Each day, set aside thirty to sixty minutes when you can work without interruption. This will give you time to read the instructions and to do the breath exercise.

As you progress through each step, you will eventually be asked to sit for one hour. Although this seems like a long time, do not feel defeated even before you attempt it. Work at your own pace. It may take a few months before you feel ready to sit for an hour. However, at some point it would be good to get past sitting for only twenty or twenty-five minutes. Longer practice sessions yield different results; you will benefit greatly if you can sit for one hour without becoming distracted. Once you realize the benefits, you might be inspired to sit for two hours.

A long-term goal is to practice breath awareness twice a day—one hour in the morning and one in the evening. This amount of time would be ideal and would give you the best results. However, for now, even twenty minutes is a great start.

By the time you complete all ten lessons you should be able to sit for one hour without any trouble. Be proud of yourself when this happens;

you will know that your mind has developed more focus, and that you have gained more equanimity.

You can follow the recommended times for sitting or challenge yourself by lengthening them. However, if you adjust the time, always remember to remain seated until the end. If you choose ten minutes, sit ten minutes. In this way you will develop self-discipline. Giving up at nine minutes would be counterproductive. It is often in the last few minutes of sitting that the best work gets accomplished—especially overcoming the habit of quitting before you are finished.

You can spread the ten lessons over a two-week period or complete a couple of lessons in one day. You might even repeat one step several times before moving to the next step. Only move forward when you feel comfortable and confident with what you are doing.

Equanimity and Focus

There is no guarantee that sitting every day for an hour or two will ensure less pain, restlessness, or agitation. You will discover that some breath awareness sessions go well while others do not. Rather than feeling disappointed, remind yourself that the goal is not to experience ongoing pain-free pleasure. Rather, the aim is to improve your ability to concentrate while developing more equanimity. Equanimity means calmly observing pleasant, neutral, and unpleasant sensations without developing craving or aversion toward them.

When you practice daily, you will find that sitting for one hour becomes easier. This achievement is not because you have less agitation or pain. Rather, you simply have developed more focus and equanimity; you can bear more physical pain than before.

Dedicated practice will lead you to experience varying degrees of concentration. These mind states can be quite profound or enjoyable. They usually result after prolonged one-pointed focus. Even a beginner may experience exquisite moments of deep concentration. When the mind is fully concentrated it sometimes reaches a mind state called *absorption*. Many of us have experienced absorption when getting 'lost' in what we are doing; for example, writing, listening to music, or painting.

When you experience perfect concentration, time seems to slow and you seem to enter into a new realm, one beyond thought. Your body feels weightless; sitting becomes effortless. Physical pain dissolves and subtle energy can be felt vibrating throughout your body. You may feel very peaceful and experience a sense of infinite space expanding inside and around you. Sometimes you may envision lights or colors, hear sounds, or experience other mental phenomenon.

Refrain from Craving

When experiencing concentrated mind states, your immediate reaction may be to prolong the experience. However, remember that your goal is to develop equanimity. It is best to acknowledge the sensation and then resume focusing on your breath. During breath awareness, pleasurable states come and go. Clinging to temporary blissful feelings defeats the goal of developing less attachment and more wisdom.

Children also experience absorption but they might not consider the feelings to be out of the ordinary. Some students describe the sensation as dizziness, light-headedness, or floating. For some children, the experience is unsettling.

When teaching breath awareness, it is important to discern whether or not a student's experience comes from concentrating or if it is a symptom of an underlying condition. A child could actually be experiencing low blood sugar, faintness, irregular heart rate, allergic reactions, or the side effects of medication.

Talking about various concentration states might cause you or a beginner student to become curious. The problem is that hearing about these pleasant or interesting experiences might make you want to seek them rather than focusing on your breath. Wanting these states becomes another distraction and is counterproductive.

Another mistake that some beginners make is to think that the experience of blissful sensations indicates that they have 'arrived' at the ultimate goal. Then when the pleasant sensations disappear, as they do after even a few minutes, the beginner may start wishing, wanting, craving, and hoping for their return. If this happens to you, acknowledge that your mind is craving and go back to observing your breath.

Progress is not measured by how many hours you can sit or by how many blissful experiences you enjoy. Rather, progress is measured by how balanced you remain. A mature student is equanimous with whatever pleasant, neutral, or unpleasant sensations manifest. A person who has mastered the mind can sit calmly through painful sessions and let nothing disturb his or her focus.

Getting up before a breath awareness session ends can become a habit. In addition, crowding the mind with thoughts while sitting can also become a habit. Our goal is to transform habits so they no longer control our behavior. If you find yourself habitually getting up or distracting yourself with thoughts, merely acknowledge what is happening and go back to focusing on the breath.

Noble Suffering

Calmly bearing discomfort or observing pleasurable feelings without attachment does not mean gritting your teeth and being a martyr. There is something called *noble suffering*—to bear pain with the wisdom and acceptance that all things of this material world are constantly changing. Noble suffering leads to detachment, wisdom, and love.

Although some breath awareness sessions are anything but blissful, know that as long as you stay focused on your breath, important transformation is taking place. When negative conditioning manifests, no matter how unpleasant, it is a sign that you are practicing correctly. Obstacles such as pain, boredom, or restlessness challenge the mind; without roadblocks to overcome or mountains to ascend, the mind could not grow strong. When irritable moments arise, see them as opportunities to develop equanimity and a noble heart.

A Wholesome Foundation Promotes Better Focus

As you work through the program, keep in mind what you do outside of your practice. Remember to perform wholesome actions to the best of your ability. Make an effort to avoid saying or doing anything that will cause your mind to become overly agitated.

If you have an unhealthy habit such as smoking or drinking, avoid it for the duration of the program. It also helps to minimize watching violent films, excessive television, or doing anything that drains your energy. As well, choose to eat healthy, natural food. Unless you are underweight, try to reduce portions especially in the evening. Doing breath awareness on an empty stomach helps deepen concentration. However, if you find yourself feeling uncomfortably full, still try to do your evening breath awareness practice. Remember that equanimity is your goal. Acknowledge your full feeling and, despite feeling uncomfortable, use the opportunity to develop equanimity.

There is More to Mind than Thought

From the time we were young we have paid a great amount of attention to the thinking side of our brains. Thinking is very useful and helps us rationalize, remember, relate, reason, relate, judge, count, deduce, and compare. The thinking brain is also enormously entertaining; the imagination creates exciting scenes and images that stir up all sorts of emotions and ideas. Thinking helps us with day-to-day activities, remembering the past, and planning the future. However, thinking can prevent us from experiencing the other more intuitive side of the brain.

Just because our intellect and imagination are engaging does not mean we have to stay trapped in them. There are other faculties of mind worth using, exploring, and experiencing. Developing concentration will enable you to direct your attention inward to discover more superior mental faculties and to awaken their latent powers. Training your attention to access these faculties is rewarding; you will realize that you are much more than you *think* you are.

Having read all the chapters to this point and having learned intellectually about the breath awareness technique, you are well prepared for the experiential stage of this path. Proceed confidently through all the steps. Know that you have embarked on what could be the most rewarding journey of your life.

STEP ONE

The Art of Breath Awareness

"My foot fell asleep. I couldn't get comfortable. My hand
was itchy. I yawned four times. My eyes were heavy.
I could hardly breathe. My thoughts took over my mind.
My head was heavy. I almost fell asleep. When my
mind wanders, I bring my focus back to my breath.
I want to keep working at it." —Marnie, Age 9

YOUR PRACTICE SESSION – STEP ONE (20 Minutes)

Breath awareness is a simple technique, but only through repetition of practice and intensity of experience can you affect real inner change. Breath awareness can restructure the brain, trigger physiological processes to enhance health, and develop a mind capable of experiencing happiness and peace. Before you embark on this transformational journey, prepare yourself both inwardly and outwardly. Be courageous and willing to walk this path alone. Not everyone is ready to look within, understand why there is discontent and disease, and find a remedy. Your partner, your children, your closest friend, and all the people you see who are suffering, may not share your enthusiasm. If you are asked to explain why you do breath awareness, or find yourself defending your beliefs in the face of skepticism, be diplomatic and empathetic of other people's opinions or feelings. Arguing may cause undue agitation and end up dampening your own inspiration to continue. Guard your innermost wish to be happy and share your aspirations with those who understand, care, and support your endeavors.

When you begin this introspective journey you are like a vulnerable sapling. Protect yourself against external forces that could undermine your growth until your roots are well-established and your purpose is clear. It is difficult to proceed confidently if friends and family misunderstand what you are doing. Be confident and stay focused on your goal. Later, when you are a mature tree sharing your shade, fruit, and beauty, others will notice your transformation and may be inspired to do the same.

There are several options to completing the ten adult breath awareness lessons. You might choose to read and perform one session each day, which will allow you to complete the program in approximately two weeks. This goal will require strong determination and a willingness to increase your sitting times to one hour over a shorter period. An even more challenging approach would be to condense the ten steps into a short span by doing two or three sessions in one day. A less demanding approach would be to do a new step at the beginning of each week, practice the suggested time for one week, and then proceed to the next step. Whichever way you choose to do the program will be beneficial.

Choose a time of day when you will be least disturbed or needed for other family responsibilities. Early in the morning or in the evening would be great if you have a busy life. You may also find time after everyone has gone to sleep, although the problem with practicing late at night is natural sleepiness. Select a quiet corner in your home where the lights can be dimmed. The area should be organized and free of distracting clutter. Ticking clocks can be annoying; use a quiet clock that has illuminated numbers visible if it is dark. After some practice you will get a sense for how much time has passed and will only have to glance at the clock now and again. Using a clock is an important part of the practice. Without a set time you would get up when sitting became uncomfortable, which would be counterproductive to developing focus.

To develop your ability to sit longer and concentrate better, practice breath awareness by sitting with your legs loosely crossed or in a kneeling position on the floor. Use a firm cushion or folded blankets high enough to prop you up and to let your knees drop down slightly. A cross-legged position creates a tripod effect and provides great stability. If this position does not work, try sitting on the edge of a chair with your feet placed flat on the floor or crossed at the ankles. Using a back support or soft couch may cause drowsiness, which makes doing breath awareness difficult. Make adjustments until you find what position works best.

If the room is cool, you may want to drape a shawl around your shoulders. Be warm, but not hot. Wrapping a shawl around you will also provide a sense of comfort and protection. Sit somewhere where insects will not bother you; compassionately remove flies, wasps, bees, mosquitoes, or other buzzing critters from the room. Close windows to minimize outside noise if the room is not too stuffy. Once you have found a comfortable sitting position on your cushion or chair, fold your hands in your lap or rest them on your knees. Whenever possible, keep your eyes closed or lowered while doing breath awareness.

Start your session with a calm and quiet mind. When ready, direct your attention to your breathing. You do not need to control your breath, breath deeply, or change your breathing in anyway. Breath awareness is not a breathing exercise. Your job is simply to observe your natural, normal breath as it is. When you inhale, feel the breath flow over the area of skin at the entrance of your nostrils or slightly above your upper lip. Be aware of its cool temperature or slight stinging inside your nose. Now be aware of your breath leaving your nose; feel its warm air flowing out and touching the small area of skin at the entrance of your nostrils. For twenty minutes remain continuously aware of your incoming and outgoing respiration softly touching your skin at the entrance of your nose and its cool or warm sensation inside your nose.

The only difficult part of breath awareness is keeping your attention continuously fixed on *feeling* the breath. Given any opportunity, your attention wanders away from your breath. You become distracted by an external event—a noise in the next room or a bird chattering outside the window. Or you start examining other things going on in your body—a numb foot, an aching back, or a rumbling stomach. Or you let your mind do what it likes to do best—think, imagine, remember, stress, hope, anticipate, doubt, analyze, and so on. Your aim in this session is to develop the ability to concentrate on feeling the breath for twenty minutes without becoming distracted. This goal may take some time to do, so for now even a few minutes is an achievement.

Until your mind becomes calm and sensitive, you might not be able to feel the breath's touch. If you cannot feel it on your skin or inside your nose, breathe harder until you can. Once you do feel your breath, go back to normal breathing and see if you can still feel it. Keep doing this until you are successful. Even if you feel nothing, if you remain focused on the area below your nose you will eventually feel the subtle, almost imperceptible, touch of air. Breath awareness requires that you observe and feel the soft touch of natural respiration. Natural breath means exactly that—your normal, ordinary, everyday breath. Sometimes your natural breath is rapid and shallow; sometimes it is long and deep. Sometimes your breathing is erratic; other times rhythmic. Sometimes your nose is stuffy and breathing is strained or noisy. The main thing to remember is that the object of focus is always your natural, normal breath, as it is, in the moment you are aware of it.

Many of us do various breath exercises like Pranayama, belly breathing, or controlled breathing to deal with pain or stress. Some of us visualize white light while we breathe or use our breath to heal and energize different parts of our body. These breathing technique are similar but not quite the same as breath awareness. To understand the difference, it is helpful to put aside the other techniques while learning breath awareness or you may start mixing techniques and compromise the results. While working through the program, it is recommended that you practice exactly as instructed. Then when you go back to other breathing techniques and exercises you will know the difference.

Breath awareness provides a way to observe your reality as it is—not the "reality" you create in your imagination. The aim is to develop the ability to observe reality objectively and without reaction. This is the reason why you do not control, slow, or change your breathing. The moment you start manipulating your breathing, you interfere with what would be happening naturally. When you objectively "watch" the breath you are actually experiencing it while being aware of it. This is a rare event. Usually we experience something while simultaneously reacting to it without much awareness. In this technique you will not be using your imagination, you will be experiencing sensation the whole time. Thoughts and imagination are also real and do exist, but they are intangible, transient, and illusionary, whereas a sensation is tangible.

For breath awareness to effectively transform deeply ingrained habits and conditioning, we need to work with actual sensations and concrete experiences. We need to feel pain, pleasure, restlessness, or irritability, or experience emotions like sadness, depression, anger, or fear in order to change our unconscious reactions to these sensations and feelings. Otherwise, we could simply imagine something like fear or pain, and imagine changing our reaction to it. This futile mind game would simply engage our fantasy, and none of our deep-rooted conditioning would manifest to give us the opportunity to change our reaction to the conditioning. Therefore, when you practice breath awareness, remember to not stay engrossed in thinking and imagination, because the technique will be less effective.

When you observe your breath, you will be continually *experiencing* your reality as it happens in the moment. Like a scientist, you will objectively examine every detail of your breath—its temperature, characteristics, rhythm, which nostril it is entering and leaving, and how it changes over the course of a sitting. The moment you manipulate or control your breathing you will no longer be observing your natural reality. When you realize that you are controlling your breath, merely acknowledge that you are controlling it and resume breathing naturally. Your aim is to become aware of your reality by feeling it. You want to experience what is going on at exactly the moment a sensation manifests. The aim is to stay alert, attentive, and connected with every sensation that arises and manifests on your skin in this limited area. This is how you consciously experience your "now" state.

To perform breath awareness, begin focusing your entire attention on a small patch of skin about one or two centimeters in diameter located directly below the nostrils and immediately above your upper lip. If you were to spread your attention to studying larger areas, you may compromise developing one-pointed focus. Your first goal is to develop a sharp and alert mind capable of examining the tiniest details of your physical reality. Although you begin by limiting your area of examination, you will learn a great deal about your mind/body phenomenon by studying this one small spot. Once your attention is sharp and focused, you will have the ability to perform a penetrating and meticulous examination of your entire physical and mental structure and experience deeper levels of your reality.

Decide how long you wish to sit for your first practice. In the beginning, it is recommended that you adhere to the suggested times. This first session is for twenty. If this seems too long, work for ten. Whether you sit for ten or twenty minutes, the important point is to remain sitting until the time is up. If you choose twenty minutes, sit twenty minutes— right down to the last second. If you choose ten minutes, sit for the full ten minutes. Glance at a clock and determine when the time will be up. Set an alarm if you like, but know that an alarm will startle you unless it is a quiet one. It is fine to open your eyes occasionally to check the time as long as it does not distract you from feeling your breath. With experience, you will be able to determine how much time has passed.

In this first breath awareness session, commit to sitting for twenty minutes. This commitment will help you develop discipline and determination. When sitting becomes uncomfortable, and it will, know that the real work has begun. Make a strong determination to sit through any discomfort, restlessness, or boredom. Persist and be rewarded. If you have pain in your legs or back, slowly shift your position. Whenever you move, move consciously so as not to overreact and break your concentration. While changing positions, continue feeling your breath. Moving your leg or foot should not interrupt your focus.

When you first start observing your breath it may be awkward to breathe naturally. It takes a bit of practice to breathe normally when observing the breath because we become self-conscious, which actually changes how we breathe. After a few breaths your attention might wander. As soon as you discover that you are thinking rather than feeling the breath, start again. Focus on the incoming breath. Focus on the outgoing breath. There is nothing more to do. You might become aware of your breath's temperature—its cool softness entering your nose and its warmth as it leaves. This is good. Feeling everything about the breath is essential to this technique. Where there is feeling there is experience and this technique is all about actual, real experience. The moment you stop feeling and get distracted in thought, the *now* experience is gone. Continue being mindful of breathing. You may start to notice the breath causing occasional itchiness or stinging—sensations manifest when the mind becomes aware of the breath touching the skin.

Be Aware of Every Breath
In this particular technique you do not follow your breath inside your body. You keep your attention fixed at all times on the small area of skin below your nose. Breath awareness is about being continuously aware of breath as it passes over this one spot. The smaller the area, the sharper your focus becomes. If you are imagining your breath entering your nose, traveling to the back of your mouth, down your throat, and then filling your chest, lungs, and stomach, you are practicing a different exercise. In breath awareness, the attention remains fixed on the small area of skin at the entrance of the nostrils. If you cannot feel your breath's delicate touch, take some harder breaths until you can. Once you detect it, resume natural, normal breathing. As long as you fix your attention on the area where you should be feeling your breath, your mind will gradually become more sensitive and alert. Soon you will be able to feel the breath ever so slightly. If the mind is preoccupied or insensitive, feeling the breath's touch will be difficult. If you do not feel its touch, that is fine, but continue focusing on the exact area of skin below your nose. You will probably feel the skin throbbing, itching, tickling, vibrating, or stinging. Although these sensations are not the touch of

breath, they will keep you focused until you do feel it. Continue concentrating on natural breathing without missing a single breath. Be aware of how many consecutive breaths you can feel before your attention wanders, but resist counting. Counting can become a distraction. Pure natural breath is all that you want to focus on. This technique does not use counting. At first, you may only be aware of five or six breaths before your mind wanders. When your mind wanders, simply bring it back to the touch of breath. Attention training happens by repetitively bringing focus back to the breath. The length of time that you focus on the breath will eventually stretch into a minute or two, and eventually you will focus for ten or fifteen minutes. Focusing purely on feeling without letting your attention wander into your imagination is difficult in the beginning, but with practice it becomes easier.

Drowsiness and fatigue can become obstacles to breath awareness. Sleepiness may simply indicate that you need more rest, but it can also be how your subconscious copes with pain, boredom, frustration, or stress. If you keep nodding off or feel overly tired, acknowledge your sleepiness, straighten your back, and take a few harder breaths. If this doesn't wake you up, open your eyes for a few minutes. If fatigue still overwhelms you, stand up, walk around, and then sit down and continue working. Remember that when you do any one of these things, stay continually focused on your incoming and outgoing breath in order to not break your concentration. Return to breath awareness and make an effort not to let one single breath go unnoticed. Now and again, however, your mind will slide back into thinking. Know that each time you start thinking or imagining, it is like landing your aircraft and postponing your journey; it will take much longer to arrive at your destination. To reach your goal—a more calm and focused mind—you must keep your attention continuously fixed on the area below your nose or slightly above your upper lip. When twenty minutes is over, resist jumping up and tending to all those tasks and duties calling for your attention. Take a minute to savor the moment, stretch your legs, and be mindful of how your body and mind feel. If you had an inattentive, irritable practice session, acknowledge how it was, and smile. Remember, whether your experience was focused or unfocused, pleasant or unpleasant, maintaining equanimity is the key to success.

TEACHER TIPS

The teacher who is indeed wise does not bid you to enter the house of his wisdom but rather leads you to the threshold of your mind. —Kahlil Gibran

Teaching Breath Awareness to Children

In each chapter, you will find *Teacher Tips* to mentor you in becoming a breath awareness teacher for children. Tips offer in-depth explanations about the technique along with strategies and approaches for delivering breath awareness lessons to children. The explanations expound on the chapter's theme, help expand intellectual understanding of the technique, and provide a map and compass for your journey.

Teacher Tips are not only written for future teachers, they are also meant to provide valuable information to augment and enhance your own practice. You might enjoy reading these tips as you work through *Your Practice* sessions.

Before any person, young or old, attempts breath awareness, there should be some degree of mental calmness. If the mind is experiencing turbulent waves on its surface, it will be difficult to see what lies beneath. Because breath awareness requires us to direct our attention inward and investigate the root cause of agitation, restlessness, and conditioned behavior, we need to start with a quiet mind. Of course, doing breath awareness will calm the most restless mind, but it will be more effective if the mind is relatively still to begin with.

To benefit from your effort, choose to do and say things in your daily life that contribute to peace and harmony. Keep in mind that there is little in life more precious than equanimity. There is no advantage to perpetuating anger or ill will, getting overly flustered, or complaining about your circumstances. What you do, what you say, and how you treat others and yourself either contribute to calmness, or stirs up agitation.

Words and actions influence our peace of mind; there is no escaping this reality. When the mind is agitated, intoxicated, dull, angry, disappointed, or excessively excited, breath awareness is difficult to do. Once we realize that it is virtually impossible to cultivate peace and happiness if we keep hurting or disturbing others, or ourselves, we will be motivated to change our ways. Many of our mind-agitating and unhealthy behaviors have become deeply ingrained, hard-to-change conditioning. Through practicing breath awareness, and becoming more conscious of our conditioning, habits gradually lose their control over us. By living a healthy and wholesome life, we not only improve our breath awareness practice, but also enjoy the long-lasting rewards of a tranquil mind.

Being the Teacher
Teachers play an essential role in the experience and success of their students. Teacher responsibilities include knowing how to perform breath awareness correctly and instructing children in easy-to-understand language. Tasks also include ensuring that children understand and follow the practical guidelines and rules of the program. Duties involve organizing a program, securing a facility, educating parents, creating application and permission forms, delivering introductory talks, and creating follow-up sessions.

When you are the teacher, you are the students' role model; everything you do or say will convey the teaching and inspire students. The vibration of your voice, your choice of words and actions, and your clarity and enthusiasm all contribute to their learning. Through your conviction in the value of the technique, you will establish an atmosphere of sincerity and respect.

Students join Mindmastery of their own volition and are generally well behaved and willing to learn. However, the technique may trigger a release of repressed behaviors or excessive restlessness. Despite children's well-intended efforts to follow the rules and practice seriously, it is not always easy to do. When a child is disruptive or disrespectful, show empathy and understanding. If a student continuously acts out, it might indicate that he or she is not inwardly ready to perform breath awareness. No matter what deeper issues are causing the outbursts, a child's mind may be simply too agitated to focus well. Should this happen, offer an activity that will help the student to calm down; for example, painting, drawing, reading, writing, or a physical exercise. To have this option available, however, you would need extra supervision.

Depending on how you have scheduled your program there may be more breaks and free-time activities, which may entail preparing healthy snacks and supervising games. Games should be non-competitive and have minimal physical contact.

Because you are established in breath awareness, you will assume leadership of the program. If other adults are assisting, however, you might be confronted with situations requiring diplomacy. Some volunteers may offer unique ideas about how to change the program, such as mixing other wholesome techniques with breath awareness. As you already understand the importance of not mixing techniques, acknowledge their ideas but politely explain that the students are simply to focus on natural respiration and nothing more. Adhere to the pure technique to prevent children from becoming confused or from minimizing the positive effects.

Adults may complain that the technique is too strict, difficult, or tedious. Their arguments might sound persuasive, but if you are established in breath awareness you will be able to stand firm. The technique is most powerful when practiced in its simple purity. Adding anything, even if the idea is wholesome, could compromise the results. Additionally, adults who volunteer should either be experienced in breath awareness or learn alongside the children.

The key to a successful program is your preparedness. You must be ready for both the practical work and, more importantly, for the inner work. Before you begin teaching, you might reflect on your motivation and your readiness. Do you feel established in the technique? Do you live a wholesome, healthy life? Do you want to give selflessly to help children?

Before you organize a group of children, determine the length of the program, secure a location, interest parents or principals in a Mindmastery program be sure to review these chapters: *You, the Teacher, Facilitating a Mindmastery Program, Student and Teacher Experience,* and *Questions and Answers* The information provided will help you to facilitate a successful program.

During the student practice sessions, you will sit in front of the group role modeling good posture. Other than explaining the technique and facilitating the lessons, one of you your primary instructions will be to remind students to bring their attention back to the breath. This will be your key line. If one or more students are disruptive, speak to them individually. Children will be sensitive to the tone of your voice—especially if experiencing agitation. The vibration of your voice will either help children calm down or fuel their frustration.

Whenever you give a prompt during a practice session, children may lose focus, become impatient, or have difficulty regaining concentration.

Try to minimize verbal interjections during practice sessions by giving instructions *before* commencing.

The Power of Breath Awareness

Breath awareness is a powerful technique that can trigger suppressed emotions such as anger, fear, or sadness. Some children avoid feeling pain by keeping themselves distracted. They might talk to themselves, act out, bite their nails, vibrate their legs, grimace, or start to sway. If you notice someone struggling, attempt to finish the session without drawing attention to him or her. Later, talk to the child privately.

Distracting the mind from feeling pain is an ingrained habit. It is how most of us avoid disturbing thoughts and painful feelings. If children are having difficulty, suggest that they do a quiet activity like drawing or reading instead. Let them know that what they're experiencing is normal and not a sign of failure or weakness. It is best if they can do an activity in another room so as not to disturb the group. To accommodate this, you will need to organize supervision.

Frequently acknowledge the children's efforts. Be patient and empathetic. Breath awareness is not a test of ability or intelligence. We should also not take their lack of focus and restlessness as a reflection of our own inadequacies. We should not express disappointment when they do not catch on immediately or live up to our expectations.

When children are working seriously, simply acknowledge that they are working properly. Extensive praise or any amount of criticism is unnecessary. This kind of acknowledgement is counterproductive. Remember, the goal is to observe reality as it is—without judgment.

About Student Instructions and Student Practice Sessions

Each chapter presents sections called *Student Instructions* and *Student Practice Sessions*. These are written in a script format that can be either be read aloud or delivered in your own words. Each session builds on the previous with slight variations. The program works best when followed one step at a time.

STUDENT INSTRUCTIONS - STEP ONE

The Art of Breath Awareness

Welcome to your first session of Mindmastery. Today you will learn a simple exercise that will improve your ability to focus while helping you learn more about your mind. The technique is *breath awareness*, and simply involves being mindful of your incoming and outgoing breath. Practicing breath awareness strengthens attention, improves focus, and develops mindmastery. Being able to focus and master your distracted, restless mind are important skills that can enhance all areas of your life including school, sports, personal activities, health, and relationships.

Working through the ten steps of Mindmastery and learning the breath awareness technique is similar to embarking on an adventure where you set out to explore an undiscovered, new world—the world inside you; the world of your mind and body. This exciting and meaningful journey will lead you to many new discoveries about your mind, thoughts, imagination, emotions, feelings, and physical reality.

Before you begin this journey, you will need a goal, a map, a compass, a seaworthy ship, and a sturdy anchor. Without these important tools, you may begin your journey only to discover that your ship is leaking, your anchor is inadequate, and that you are drifting in the wrong direction. To prepare yourself, the first thing is to be clear about your goals. Why work through this challenging program and learn breath awareness? The goal of learning breath awareness is to become more peaceful, focused, and joyful. You also want to know yourself deeply and become self-aware. Without self-awareness, without mastery over the reactive, restless mind, we can never be truly happy. Happiness is your journey's destination.

To succeed at reaching your destination, a sea-worthy, stable ship is required, one that is strong and sound. This ship is your mind. You create a sound, calm mind by the actions that you perform in your daily life. To create a calm mind, you must ensure that whatever you do or say, how you treat others or yourself is helpful and healthy. To ensure that your mind-ship is strong, try to refrain from doing anything that harms others or yourself. Wholesome actions will become your anchor in a storm; your foundation for focus; and your insurance that breath awareness will lead you to more joy. Without a firm foundation and a sturdy anchor, your ship may drift away. Make your anchor strong by refraining from unwholesome actions or doing anything that will agitate your mind. Breath awareness is too difficult to do if your mind is overly disturbed. For this reason, refrain from doing or saying anything that will compromise your focus training.

Your map will be the lessons; your compass will be your intuition. You will hear many instructions and ideas, but do not accept these as true. Only accept things as true after you have experienced them for yourself. The journey is about discovering your own truths. Your intuition and intelligence will guide you along and keep you on the right track. Always follow your sense of what is right; this will lead you to the achievement of your goals.

Now that you have a goal, ship, map, compass, and anchor, it is time to set off on an introspective journey and explore your inner world. To perform breath awareness, resume a comfortable sitting position. You may sit cross-legged or in a kneeling position and use a cushion or folded blanket for support. If this is uncomfortable or inconvenient, you may sit in your desk or on a chair. Whatever position you choose, your back, spine, and neck are aligned and straight. There is no need to tighten your muscles or strain; be relaxed, but do not slump over. You can remove your glasses as the exercise does not require any reading or looking around at things in the room. If you are close to your neighbor, or if your knee is touching someone's cushion, allow yourself more room. You do not want to disturb anyone while practicing.

If you are sitting on a chair, sit on its edge and try not to lean back even when you get tired. If you lean back you might get sleepy and the muscles in your back will not get stronger. Your hands can be resting in your lap or on your knees. No matter what sitting position you choose, make sure to keep your back straight. When we do breath awareness, we stay silent because it helps us pay attention to what is going on in our minds. We usually try to keep our eyes closed, but if you have trouble closing your eyes you may look down at your hands or a spot on the floor.

Now let us begin learning how to do the breath awareness exercise. Start by directing your attention to your natural, normal breathing. Feel your breath as you breathe in. Do you feel the touch of breath just at the entrance of your nostrils? Do you feel the breath inside your nose? Is it cool? Does it sting? Is it itchy? Now feel your breath as you breathe out. Do you feel its temperature? Do feel it touch your skin ever so softly? Continue watching each breath as you inhale and as you exhale. Every breath is important. Try not to miss a single breath.

Always breathe through your nose, not through your mouth unless you have a stuffy nose. Breathe as you would normally breathe if you were not thinking about it. There is no need to change how you breathe by slowing your breath or taking deep breaths. All you have to do is breathe naturally. If you have been running around, your normal breathing may feel fast. If you have been sitting quietly, your normal breathing may be soft and shallow. The exercise is to feel your normal, ordinary, natural breath.

If you cannot feel your soft breath, try to fix your attention either inside your nose or on the area below your nostrils until you do feel something. If you must, take a few harder breaths so you can feel it, then go back to breathing naturally. Every time you realize that you have stopped feeling your breath and that you are thinking or imagining things, acknowledge, *I have lost my focus* and resume breath awareness. You do not have to sit perfectly still, and if you are uncomfortable, move your legs or body just enough to relieve the pain or pressure. Move slowly, though, while continuing to feel your breath. In this way, you will not interrupt your breath awareness practice and will continue to strengthen your concentration.

For the full ten minutes that you will be working in this first session, remember to keep your attention focused on your incoming and outgoing breath, feeling its touch below the entrance of your nose or inside your nose. Do not control your breathing in any way. Become a scientist who has been given a research assignment to study the natural characteristics of breath. While you are sitting, you can ask, *What is my breath doing right now? What is its temperature? How does it feel?* Have you all understood how to do breath awareness? Are there any questions? We will dim the lights to help you keep your eyes closed and to avoid distraction. Are you comfortable? Is your back straight? Relax your shoulders. We will practice breath awareness for ten minutes. Let us begin with a calm and quiet mind.

STUDENT PRACTICE SESSION (10 Minutes)

Two-minute Silent Practice

Sit up straight and relax your shoulders. Keep your chin tucked in slightly and your hands folded in your lap. Focus your entire attention at the base of your nose and feel your incoming breath touch the skin in this area. Now, breathe out and feel the outgoing breath touch the skin at the entrance of your nose. Now, breathe in. If you cannot feel the breath in this area try to feel it inside your nose.

If you lose focus and your mind wanders, acknowledge, *Oh my mind has wandered*, and bring your attention back to the touch of breath. Has your body become uncomfortable or tired? Acknowledge, *Oh my body is uncomfortable*, and bring your focus back to your breath. Every time you lose concentration return to feeling your breath. If you need to change your position, change slowly without letting one single breath escape your attention.

Six-minute Silent Practice

Feel the breath as it comes in. Examine it. Is it cooler coming in? Feel the breath as it goes out. Examine it again. Is it warmer going out? Have you opened your eyes and become distracted? Are you thinking about something? Are your thoughts jumping around? This is the natural tendency of an untrained mind.

Close your eyes. Sit erect and refocus your attention on your breath. Keep your back straight. Feel your breath as it comes in and touches the area of skin at the entrance of your nose. Is it a long breath? Is it a short breath? Is it a deep breath? Is it shallow?

Two-minute Silent Practice - Session Concludes

You may open your eyes and change positions so that you are comfortable. However, do not lie down. It is time for a story.

RESTLESS GETS TRAINED

Once upon a time there was a boy named Jay. While playing in his backyard, Jay peeked through a hole in the fence. This was not the first time that he watched Fetchit Sam, his neighbor's big friendly dog. He watched while Fetchit Sam ran to retrieve a Frisbee and bring it back to his owner. Jay admired Fetchit Sam and thought, *If only I could have a well-trained dog, I would be so happy.* That night, Jay mustered up his courage and asked his father, "Please Dad, please may I have a puppy?" His father answered, "Puppies are fun, but they require a lot of attention to train properly." Jay pleaded, "Please Dad, I promise to train the puppy every day!"

A while later, Jay and his father visited the animal shelter and after looking at many dogs, found the most rambunctious, lively puppy in the whole world. It was racing around in circles, jumping over its water bowl, and rolling over and over. "Woof! Woof!" barked the puppy, which in English means, "Pick me! Pick me!" Jay fell instantly in love with the puppy and looked up to his father who smiled and said, "What will you name him?" Jay grinned from ear to ear and said, "Restless." Jay picked up wriggly Restless and brought him home that very same day.

The next morning, when Jay awoke, Restless was gone. Jay heard some crashing and looked out the window. "Oh no!" he cried. What did he see? Garbage strewn all over the lawn, his running shoe chewed in half, a scratch on Dad's cool Masarati, and a half-eaten birthday cake. Oh, that's right, today was his birthday.

"Happy Birthday Jay!" congratulated his father while surveying the yard. "I guess today is also Training Restless Day." Jay was angry at Restless and was about to shout. Then he remembered that Restless was just a puppy. He went outside calling, "Here Restless. Come to me." However, the puppy was too busy digging a hole in the lawn and burying his running shoe. Over and over again, Jay gently called his puppy. At last, Restless returned. "Good boy!" Jay rewarded his puppy with a hug. Restless licked Jay's face and then wriggled and wiggled until he got free. Fetchit Sam started barking next door. Restless raced to the fence. "Woof! Woof!" What a racket their barking made! Jay called Restless back. This time it only took two tries. "Good boy. Now sit! Stay!" But Restless didn't like to sit still. He jumped up, knocked Jay over, and started licking his face. Again, Jay commanded, "Sit!" Finally, after twenty tries, Restless sat still.

Jay continued to patiently train Restless everyday, dreaming that one day his puppy would grow up and become a Seeing Eye dog. Because Restless was so well trained, this is exactly what happened. Restless became a dependable Seeing Eye dog and helped lead blind people. Jay was proud of Restless and was happy to see the rewards of all his efforts.

Your untrained attention, like the young puppy Restless, likes to jump playfully from one thought to the next always looking for something interesting. The secret to training your puppy dog mind is to patiently and persistently, over and over again, call your restless attention back to your breath. This is how you succeed in developing stronger attention.

Student Journal

You have worked seriously in your first Mindmastery session. You have learned how to do breath awareness properly. Keep in mind that focusing is a difficult thing to learn. Even adults find breath awareness challenging. Do not feel disappointed if you could only focus for a minute or two. Even if all you did today was notice the touch of your breath below your nose, it was a great first step!

You definitely started to train your attention muscles to work for you and you may already feel less restless and more focused. Some of you may even have discovered, for the first time, how your thoughts jump around and how you can bring them back at will.

It is now time to express your experiences in your journal. Begin by writing everything you discovered today. You may convey your findings in a story, poem, or picture. Whichever way you choose, describe all the details of what happened while sitting still. Do not worry about spelling mistakes or if you cannot draw exactly what is in your mind. Be patient with yourself if you have not yet mastered the breath awareness technique. We are all just beginners and it takes time to learn this challenging skill.

You may go quietly and begin working in your journals. For the first fifteen minutes we will work in silence, which will allow you time to express your thoughts. After journal time we can share our discoveries and stories.

CHECK-IN

Check-in questions help you, the adult, reflect on your experiences during *Your Practice* sessions.

- Were you able to feel the breath as it passed over the area of skin just below your nose and above your upper lip?

- Could you stay with the touch of breath without your mind wandering into your thoughts for at least a few minutes?

- When your body became restless, were you able to bring your attention back to your breath? Did you notice your body calm down?

- When your mind wandered, did you notice if you were thinking about the past or the future? How long did it take to realize that your mind had wandered before you brought your attention back to your breath?

- Could you sit for at least ten or fifteen minutes without moving your position? If you had to move, could you still stay focused on your breath while moving?

- Did you notice any physical changes when your mind became quiet? Could you remain sitting still, objectively observing the touch of breath, despite feeling pain or discomfort?

Continuation of Practice Tip: During the rest of the day, be aware of your breath while working, walking, cooking, doing dishes, showering, watching television, or listening to someone. At night, before falling asleep, feel your breath for five minutes. Then, when you wake up, feel your breath for five minutes. Although your experience may not be as focused or intense as during your breath awareness sittings, continuation of practice is the secret of success! Remember, when it comes to building brain networks and influencing physiological processes, intensity and repetition of the exercise affects greater change.

STEP TWO

Learning through Experience

"It wasn't that hard, actually it was easy. I yawned fourteen
times. I know that because I counted, but each time I got back to
my breath. Some of my sensations are the cold feelings when
you breathe in and the hot feeling when you breathe out."
—Andrew, Age 9

YOUR PRACTICE — STEP TWO (30 Minutes)

Your second breath awareness practice will be for thirty minutes. Resume a comfortable position and keep your back and neck straight, yet relaxed. Begin with a calm and peaceful mind; let nothing disturb your tranquility. Close your eyes and fix your attention on the incoming and outgoing breath as it touches the small area below your nose. In this session, you will try to stay focused on this limited area just outside the entrance of your nostrils.

Remember that the object of focus is your natural, ordinary breath. Be mindful of your breath as it is in this moment. Is it soft? Is it quiet? Is it warm? Is it irregular? Is it deep? It makes no difference what kind of breath you are experiencing or whether it is slow, fast, deep, or long. The aim of your practice is to observe your natural breath and to feel the sensation that it creates on your skin, without controlling or manipulating it.

In this session, you will learn how to sharpen your focus. One-pointed focus is an excellent tool for performing a precise and penetrating examination of your breath. To investigate your reality, you should have a good instrument to work with.

To improve your focus, narrow your attention to observing a small one-centimeter spot below your nostrils. When you breathe in, be mindful of everything transpiring on this small spot. Determine the exact moment that your incoming breath touches this spot, and then continue observing as the incoming breath passes over this spot. After you have completed your in-breath, see if you can determine the exact moment when you no longer feel any breath. This will be the moment just before you start breathing out.

While exhaling, again fix your attention on the small spot below your nose. Observe the outgoing breath in the same manner, being mindful of when it first touches the skin. Continue observing the breath passing over this spot. Determine the exact moment when there is an absence of breath on your skin before you start breathing in again. This close examination will let you experience the beginning, middle, and end of every inhalation and the beginning, middle, and end of every exhalation. Such examination sharpens the mind and awakens insight into the nature of experience and sensation. Experience is always connected to some kind of sensation. When you do not feel anything, you cannot experience. Experience is the root of all knowledge so, as you can see, becoming conscious of sensation is the beginning of real self awakening.

Whenever your mind wanders and you start thinking, acknowledge that your mind has wandered and that you have lost your focus. Then, refocus your attention on the incoming and outgoing breath. Repeatedly bringing your attention back to the breath trains the mind in much the same way as one would train any muscle. When other sensations in or on your body other than those felt directly below your nose distract your attention, acknowledge that you have lost focus and then resume breath awareness.

If you become overwhelmed, agitated, or distracted by a common hindrance such as sensual desire, anger, drowsiness, restlessness, or doubt, acknowledge that you are agitated and then narrow your focus to an even smaller area. Working in this manner, continue your session until thirty minutes has passed. Try to enjoy the moment rather than jumping up from your sitting. After, you may wish to reflect on your *Check-in* questions.

TEACHER TIPS

The only source of knowledge is experience. —Albert Einstein

Facilitating Experiential Learning

Your Mindmastery program should be well underway and by now most of your students will be familiar with the breath awareness technique and feel comfortable with what they are doing. If this is your first course, there may be many things going on in your mind when you are trying to do breath awareness. You might feel disorganized and unfocused. Facilitating a course, keeping everyone on track, addressing the concerns of parents and children, and dealing with your own feelings might cause you to become restless or distracted. You may worry that your agitation will spill over and affect the children's concentration.

If your mind becomes distracted, acknowledge your lack of focus and continue doing the best you can. To be more inwardly prepared, practice breath awareness before teaching others even if it means waking up earlier or ensuring that you had a good session the night before. This approach will promote your equanimity and help you to fulfill your responsibilities with a calm mind.

Learning breath awareness can only be done through one's own experience. Keeping this fact in mind is important. As teacher, your aim is to simply facilitate a breath awareness experience in children. One way to do this is to minimize the time spent giving instructions, explaining things, or letting the children spend the time engaged in conversation.

Although instructions are very important to ensure that students know what they are to do, keep your explanations clear and brief. If you hear yourself philosophizing, moralizing, or rambling you will probably lose their attention. There is nothing that cannot be learned from direct experience, therefore the sooner a child can get to the practical work the better.

On this path, self-knowledge and wisdom are gained through doing the exercises and experiencing all sensations whether painful, pleasurable, or neutral. This understanding will help to facilitate experience, rather than merely intellectualizing and talking about it.

STUDENT INSTRUCTIONS – STEP TWO

Learning through Experience

Welcome to your second Mindmastery session. Despite feeling restless, you have all worked properly by staying focused on your breath, and bringing your attention back to the breath when your mind wandered. Let us review what you have learned so far.

You first applied to this Mindmastery program because you were curious and maybe thought that it would be good to improve your concentration skills and to strengthen your mind. Then, you listened to an introduction about wholesome conduct. This talk explained how your behavior, words, and actions directly affect your ability to concentrate. You learned that acting in ways that do not harm you or anyone else helps you do breath awareness well. Wholesome conduct creates a solid foundation for developing focus.

In your last session, you were taught how to perform the breath awareness technique. You learned how to sit erect with your back straight and eyes closed, and to fix your attention on your breath. You calmed your mind enough to feel the breath's touch on a small area at the base of your nose. You examined your breath to see if it was short, long, cool, or warm. These exercises taught you about your mind. You learned that your mind is restless and has difficulty staying focused only on breath, and that it keeps getting distracted. You learned how to bring your attention back to the breath when this happens.

You learned how to sit still despite feeling uncomfortable, bored, or restless. You also learned how to change your sitting position without losing your focus. As you can see, you have already learned many important things.

Let us now begin our second breath awareness session. Remember to keep your back straight and your shoulders relaxed. If you are wearing glasses, remove them. Place your hands in your lap or on your knees. Close your eyes. We will be sitting for fifteen minutes.

STUDENT PRACTICE SESSION (15 Minutes)

Five-minute Silent Practice

Feel your natural breath as you inhale. Feel your natural breath as you exhale. Feel your breath touch the small area of skin just below your nose. Keep your entire attention fixed on feeling your natural, normal, ordinary breath.

Do not control your breath. Do not take deeper breaths. Do not hold your breath. You are observing your breath however it is in the moment. Be like a scientist studying the characteristics of breath. Is your breath warm? Is it cool? Is it soft, deep, shallow, or fast? Your job is to observe objectively what is happening with your breath.

Five-minute Silent Practice

If your mind has wandered, acknowledge if your attention has wandered, and if it has, then bring your attention back to your breath. Examine your breath in the moment. If your breathing is soft; acknowledge that it is soft. If your breath is shallow; acknowledge that it is shallow. Is your breath coming in through the right nostril? Just be aware that it is coming in through the right nostril. Is your breath coming in through the left nostril? Be aware that it is coming in through the left nostril. Is your breath entering through both nostrils? Just be aware. If you cannot feel which nostril your breath is coming through, take some harder breaths. Once you feel which nostril the air is passing through, resume quiet normal breathing.

Five-minute Silent Practice - Session Concludes

Good. You can now open your eyes. If you wish to change positions and make yourself more comfortable, you are free to do so. You have all worked well. It is time for a story.

THE STUDENT AND THE PEANUT

Once upon a time there was an ambitious, young biology student. She went to her teacher and said, "Sir, I want to learn everything you know. Please put me to work." The teacher smiled and placed a peanut on the counter. "You can start by examining this peanut. Make a report about everything you find." Then the professor left her alone.

The student looked at the peanut and started taking notes. There was nothing particularly interesting about the peanut. It was just an ordinary, normal peanut like so many she had seen before. She wrote, "The peanut has a yellow-brown casing. Its oblong shape has two bulges at either end separated with a narrow waist. Its outer shell has ridges crisscrossing one end to the other and its total length measures three centimeters." Satisfied with her work, she waited for her teacher to return.

After a while, she felt bored and restless. With nothing to do, she picked up the peanut and rolled it between her fingers while staring at the clock. Then she got up and went to look for her professor. As he was nowhere to be found, she returned to her desk and gazed at the peanut. A couple of hours passed and getting hungry, she went for lunch. When she returned she impatiently stared at the useless peanut feeling angry with her teacher. In order to kill time, the student started counting the ridges that ran vertically down the peanut's shell. Then she counted the ridges running horizontally. This completed, she measured the circumference of each bulge and then drew the peanut from all perspectives. When she drew the ridges, she realized that the shape between each ridge varied in size and depth. One end of the peanut was pointy; the other end was flat. After making these discoveries, the teacher finally returned. Excitedly, the student listed off her findings. The professor listened and then commented, "Everyone knows those things. Keep looking until you see something new."

Again, the student started examining the peanut. This time, she split it open and noted two oblong nuts covered with a fragile brown skin. They lay slightly touching each other in the shell. The interior shell was gray with speckled black and red spots. Its delicate cellular lining comprised a layer of woven fibers. The more she observed, the more interesting details came to her attention. She was proud of her discoveries and knew they would earn her praise and a good mark. However, when the professor returned and reviewed her notes, he shook his head, "Is this all you have found?"

The discouraged student spent the next three days studying the peanut. The more that she examined it, the more details revealed themselves. With renewed energy and interest, she dissected the peanut part-by-part. She peeled back the skins, split open each nut, and noted a dividing line etched into their centers. She crushed one of the nuts between her fingers until oil seeped out. She tasted the oil and noted a pleasant flavor. Next, she tasted the outer shell and found it dry and bitter. Her list of observations grew longer and longer. Just when she thought that she had discovered everything there was to know about the peanut, she placed a fragment of the peanut under a high-powered microscope and discovered countless more characteristics. She examined its cells and molecular structures. Breaking these down more, she discerned various biochemical substances. This led her to discovering atoms, protons, neutrons, and electrons orbiting in empty space. She suddenly realized that the peanut was comprised of moving subatomic particles and energy, and was not static matter, as she had once believed it to be.

Through rigorous examination of the peanut, the student's mind grew keen; she could see the subtlest nuances; her attention was highly focused; her examination methods were disciplined; and her interest in peanuts grew passionate. What had once seemed ordinary became extraordinary. She no longer found the peanut boring; she no longer felt restless and impatient. Suddenly she understood what she had learned – the art of meticulous and patient observation. She gratefully thanked her professor and continued using these skills for the rest of her life becoming one of the most prominent biologists of her time.

In the same way this student became an expert observer, you also are becoming an expert observer of your breath. You have already noticed many details such as where breath touches your skin; which nostril it enters and leaves; how the breath's temperature changes, how deep, shallow, long, or rhythmic it is. You have also observed how doing breath awareness calms your mind. You have experienced how your calm mind makes your body calm. You have noticed how your restless thoughts make you feel restless. All these observations are valuable. As you continue practicing breath awareness, you will continue to discover many more things about yourself.

Student Journal

During this sitting, you examined every detail about your breath and by doing so, you sharpened your attention. Now, like a scientist, write a list of all your observations. What sensations did the breath create? Was your breathing shallow, deep, long, or short? Did its temperature change? Did you breathe in through both nostrils or just one? How did practicing breath awareness affect your state of mind? Could you bring your attention back to your breath when your mind wandered? You may prefer drawing your observations or putting them into a story.

CHECK-IN

- Was sitting easier or more difficult this time? Could you sit for the full thirty minutes?

- Could you feel the touch of your breath? Could you observe the start, middle, and end of each incoming breath? Could you observe the start, middle, and end of each outgoing breath?

- Did you notice the difference in temperature when you were breathing in and when you were breathing out? Were there changes in your breathing rhythm? Did you notice if the air was coming in through one nostril or both nostrils?

- Did you feel overly sleepy? Sleepiness may not be from lack of sleep, rather an unconscious defense against stress. If you were sleepy, remember to take a few hard breaths then resume normal breathing.

- Did you notice a change in your physical feelings after about twenty minutes of sitting? What were the changes?

- Did you notice if your thoughts wandered to past events? Did you notice if your thoughts started to ponder the future?

- Did you sometimes lose your focus and start thinking about a series of events, almost like a story?

- Have you noticed that you have begun to think twice about doing unhealthy things such as eating too much or eating the wrong food?

- Did any of the following hindrances prevent you from focusing on your breath?

    1. *Sense Desire*—Wanting to feel better or experience a pleasant sensation, wanting something good to happen.

    2. *Ill Will or Aversion*—Wanting pain to go away, feeling angry with yourself or others, resenting someone.

3. *Laziness* and *Drowsiness*—Feeling mentally sluggish or lethargic, falling asleep to avoid focusing on or dealing with issues.

4. *Restlessness* and *Remorse*—An unsettled mental state, feeling guilty, wishing you had done things differently.

5. *Doubt*—Not believing that you can perform the work, thinking that nothing you do will help, lack of self-confidence, feeling defeated.

When you notice any one of these five hindrances, smile. It indicates that the technique is working and that your subconscious negative conditioning is manifesting. Once you become conscious of a mind state, you have an opportunity to investigate its root cause, namely its underlying sensation. You also have an opportunity to practice objective, non-reaction toward this mind state, which helps you change ingrained and unconscious reactive habit-patterns.

Continuation of Practice Tip: The next time you are overwhelmed with a feeling of depression, anger, hopelessness, worry, or doubt, practice breath awareness. It is often very difficult to sit calmly and to focus on your breath when negative emotions overwhelm you, but if you can practice long enough even though it feels as though nothing is changing, you may be surprised by how much better you feel after a session.

STEP THREE

Mastering the Habit-mind

"I have noticed that since we started Mindmastery
I have stopped chewing my nails and it helps me fall
asleep at night. I also find it frustrating when
other people are bullying." —Marissa, Age 9

YOUR PRACTICE SESSION - STEP THREE (45 Minutes)

In this session you will be sitting forty-five minutes. Practicing breath awareness for such a long period requires *strong determination*. Make a commitment to sit for the whole session. Remember to start with a calm and peaceful mind. Let nothing disturb you. These are precious minutes—use them wisely.

For the entire time, you will be paying closer attention to the touch of breath. Continue focusing on the area just below the entrance of your nose and slightly above your upper lip. Then, isolate an even smaller spot where your breath flows over your skin and keep your attention directed on this spot. The smaller the area, the sharper your attention will become.

Examine your breath as you did in the previous session. Be mindful of the beginning, continuation, and end of your incoming breath experience. Then be mindful of the beginning, continuation, and end touch of your outgoing breath. Take note if the breath is long or short. Acknowledge if the breath is deep or shallow. Reflect on the moment-by-moment changes in your experience of breath. Notice exactly when the feeling is detected. Notice how it lingers. Notice exactly when it fades. One moment you are experiencing the breath's reality, the next it is gone. Reality is experience. Being aware of the experience is being aware of your present reality.

The more subtle your breath, the more sensitive your mind becomes. Sometimes your breath will become so subtle you will not feel it. When this happens, just take a few harder breaths until you do feel the air touching your skin. After taking these harder breaths, always return to natural breathing.

Unless there is an emergency, let nothing interrupt your sitting. Stay seated until the time is up. If you feel pressure or strain in your legs, move to another position, but move slowly while keeping your attention fixed on your breath. When the time is up, you might like to reflect on the questions in your *Check-in*.

TEACHER TIPS

*Freedom is found in the choiceless awareness of our
daily existence and activity.* —Krishnamurti

Equanimity is the Goal

There are countless ways to calm our restless, agitated minds. We can listen to soothing music, walk in nature, read inspirational books, paint, or do a quiet activity. Some of us use natural herbs or medications to calm our nerves; while others go to the beach, suntan, or relax by the pool. Breath awareness also offers an effective way to calm restlessness; however, there is a fundamental difference between doing breath awareness and relaxing activities. Reading or painting are enjoyable and help to quiet restlessness, but may only calm the surface of the mind and provide temporary relief. If our aim is to experience long-lasting peacefulness, we have to heal agitation at its source.

Breath awareness can heal the deeper levels of mind provided it is practiced properly, continuously, and with sufficient intensity. Exercising equanimity toward unpleasant sensations helps to change unhealthy conditioning that caused our agitation in the first place. To become deeply peaceful, the mind must be free from conditioned behaviors and mental impurities such as anger, selfishness, intolerance, fear, resent, or greed.

Let us try to understand how equanimous observation of sensations caused by breath can help clear out mental impurities. When doing breath awareness, your attention stays exclusively focused on feeling. It does not dwell in the imagination. As mentioned earlier, the attention can do only one thing at one time; either it is feeling or it is thinking. Keeping attention fixed on *feeling* breath, prevents it from wandering into the imagination where it becomes distracted with thinking.

When a repressed or unconscious state begins to surface, you often feel uncomfortable or agitated. However, if you keep your attention focused and not let it wander, the surfacing mind state has no alternative but to manifest as a physical sensation. Ignoring the discomfort can cause the unpleasant sensation to intensify and you might feel more heat, strain, pain, or numbness.

Once a sensation manifests, whether it is pleasurable or painful, you have a tangible object to work with—namely a sensation. For example, if your back aches you will feel sensations of heat, strain, throbbing, or pressure. If boredom manifests, you may feel sensations of irritability and stress. Even though your mind has everything to do with triggering these sensations, you cannot heal, eradicate, or transform mental states if they remain abstract, intellectual concepts.

Whenever we experience physical discomfort, we usually try to get rid of the pain. This reaction is instinctual. We may take painkillers, switch on the television, go on a walk, or text a few friends. If external distractions are unavailable, we can avoid feeling pain by escaping into our imagination and thoughts.

When doing breath awareness, you do not let yourself become distracted. Instead, you embrace sensation, whether it is pleasurable or painful. By objectively observing sensation, and not reacting to it as you normally would, you stop your conditioned habit. When you lose your focus and start thinking again, you will notice that these unpleasant sensations diminish slightly. When you go back to feeling your breath, these unpleasant sensations will once again intensify. This feels more uncomfortable, but it is a good thing because you can continue your work to develop equanimity.

As long as you continue focusing on breath, surfacing unconscious states will trigger a variety of sensations including restlessness, trembling, sweating, numbness, heaviness, pain, irritability, fatigue, frustration, doubt, anger, boredom, fear, and sometimes even sensual or sexual feelings. When you become conscious of these manifesting sensations, simply acknowledge them and resume feeling the touch of respiration. The aim of this technique is to experience whatever sensation arises and not react to it.

Using distraction to escape pain is a deeply ingrained habit. That is why, for some, breath awareness seems counter-intuitive. After all, since birth, we have been conditioned to believe that pain is life threatening and must be done away with immediately. This does make sense, but instincts do not take into account that when we get rid of controlling habits, we become happier human beings.

The Pivotal Moment of Choice

The very moment that you become conscious of a painful, pleasant, or neutral sensation, make a choice not to react. This choice is pivotal to changing unwanted habits and rewiring the brain. Instead of impulsively reacting to painful sensation, it is better to—stop, look, and not react. By doing this, you begin to change your ingrained conditioned response. Choosing not to react is the mental training that breaks addictive patterns. However, saying no to a habit infuriates the habit-mind and it often rebels by intensifying unpleasant sensations. To illustrate this, just imagine what would happen if you had a habit of smoking and refused the urge to smoke—the urge would become unbearable.

When a sensation becomes unbearable, exercise more self-discipline to keep your focus fixed on feeling breath. Exercising equanimity toward unpleasant, pleasant, and neutral sensations triggers an amazing process called *mind purification*. Mind purification happens when you calmly observe uncomfortable sensations and refrain from reacting. The longer you stay calm, the more painful sensations dissipate. When the pain is gone, you will also have changed your habit response it. By continuously exercising equanimity toward unpleasant sensations, you systematical weaken your ingrained habits and clear your mind of negative states. A pure, uncontaminated mind enjoys more calmness and joy.

Calmness Doesn't Last Forever

Breath awareness helps you to be calm; but more importantly it helps you to develop *equanimity*. Why is equanimity so important? Because when calmness evaporates, as it will, you can accept that it is gone and remain balanced. Equanimity is the ability to observe your changing mind/body phenomenon without developing craving or aversion toward any particular experience. When your students start losing their cool and complaining about restlessness, aches, or boredom, explain that the aim of breath awareness is to develop equanimity, not to sustain pleasurable feelings. As well, explain how physical discomfort provides opportunity to change unhealthy habits.

Nothing lasts forever. When you are calm, you may want the feeling of calmness to stay. Nevertheless, even calmness is a conditioned state. Calmness depends on a particular set of circumstances; circumstances that are bound to change. Although you enjoy feeling serene and peaceful, try not to become attached to these temporary states.

Many of us appear calm, composed, and happy, but have deep-rooted agitation brewing within. Even if we succeed in suppressing unhappiness, we are still susceptible to unhappy states overpowering us. When our defenses are down, when tired, or when facing a crisis, suppressed states may rear up and evaporate our serenity. Negative states that you thought no longer bothered you, like jealousy, resentment, prejudice, or depression, can stay buried in your unconscious for years. When you practice breath awareness, you encourage these states to surface and manifest as sensations.

Transforming Habits

Breath awareness can help to break unhealthy habits or unwanted behaviors. A habit is a recurrent, often unconscious pattern of behavior that is acquired through frequent repetition. These repeated behaviors are usually formed from either avoiding an unpleasant sensation or doing something that creates a pleasant sensation. Over our evolution as a species, we have formed many behaviors that promote basic survival. However, habits can easily become addictions to particular stimuli compromising our health and happiness.

We develop a habit when we feel pain or discomfort and reach for a substance or perform a behavior that relieves us of this discomfort. For example, when we are bored, we may eat comfort food; when depressed we may drink alcohol. Some ingrained behaviors include how we treat others or ourselves, how we think, and how we react emotionally to a situation. If we repeat behaviors, our brain circuitry is wired in that particular way. When the brain's circuitry and neural network establishes a fixed pattern of reacting to a particular stimulus or situation, behavior becomes automatic, instinctive, or unconscious.

Once brain wiring is fixed, the habit happens more or less on its own without much thinking or effort. To change or eradicate a habit, we must undo this established circuitry. This requires retraining the brain, specifically by stopping a habitual response to a particular sensation. To do this, we must first recognize the sensation triggering the response. Then we must refrain from doing what we normally do. If we repeat this enough times, we eventually change or modify the fixed wiring. Every time we practice breath awareness, consciously feel a sensation, and do not react to it, we are rewiring our brain. If we continue not reacting, the habit response weakens.

If eradicating habits were easily accomplished, none of us would suffer addictions. However, breaking a habit is difficult; whenever we try, our habit-mind rebels like a spoiled child. It is the nature of a habit obstinately to repeat what it has always done. For example, imagine that your foot gets itchy while doing breath awareness. Your usual habit would be to scratch it. However, you refrain from doing this and continue focusing on your breath. By exercising equanimity toward the unpleasant itch, three things may happen. One, the itchiness may diminish; two, you stay focused and it does not bother you; three, the itchiness intensifies. No matter which one of these possibilities occurs, by not reacting, your habit of impulsively scratching an itch weakens. Once you develop your capacity to break a small, harmless habit, you will develop the ability to break serious ones.

The Impermanence of Reality

Practicing breath awareness causes the mind to become exceptionally sensitive. Eventually, you will feel subtle energy vibrating throughout your entire body. When you experience your rapidly changing physiology, you experience who and what you really are. Realizing that you are a mass of moving and vibrating matter helps to dissolve your conditioned belief that you are a permanent and solid entity.

To the human eye, a candle's flame appears to be the same flame it was when it started burning. What you are actually seeing, though, is an entirely different flame every second. In the same way, you perceive your body as a solid structure. If you observed your body under a microscope, however, you would see tremendous cellular activity and movement. Like the flame, your body is an entirely different body every second. Because of the rapidity of physiological change and the hard to see molecular activity, you believe that you are the same person you were a minute ago. Perhaps the only thing that stays fixed is your self-concept—intellectual memories of who you think you are. Although we all rely on our self-concept to help us relate and function in the world, it can become an obstacle to freedom. When you experience yourself perpetually changing, the experience of change lessens your attachment to your self-concept or ego.

Living in the Now

When teaching breath awareness, you will be constantly reminding your students to either "watch" their breath or "feel" it. Watch means to be mindful and attentive of the breath; while feel means to feel the soft, warm, subtle sensation caused by breath touching the skin. Both words mean to be aware of the breath, but refer to slightly different ways of being aware and seeing.

After a few sessions, children become skilled at experiencing the sensation of breath exactly when it happens. They experience how it is virtually impossible to feel breath while the attention is focused on thoughts. It becomes clear that the attention cannot be in two places at once. When feeling, the attention cannot be thinking; when thinking, the attention cannot be feeling. Upon closer examination, you and your students will discover that attention actually jumps back and forth from feeling to thinking with such rapidity it seems as though thinking and feeling occur simultaneously.

We can go through an entire day unaware of our sensations, yet sensations influence most of our decisions. To illustrate, think about driving a car for hours while avoiding dangerous situations, judging distances, speeding up, slowing down, turning, and stopping. When you arrive home, you might not even consider the sensations that governed your driving decisions. If you spent your day unconscious of sensations, you will probably feel excessively tired by night. Your sleep may be restless. Your dreams may be troubled. The more you are aware of sensations throughout the day, the less tired you will be by night.

STUDENT INSTRUCTIONS - STEP THREE

Mastering the Habit-mind

Welcome to your third Mindmastery session. Each one of you has been working seriously and most of you now understand how to do breath awareness correctly. Your last practice may have been difficult. It is common to feel more restlessness, agitation, or boredom at this stage. Your head, arms, legs, stomach, feet, or back may have felt sore and uncomfortable, which then distracted you from focusing. You may have started thinking about ways to get rid of the pain. Be assured that increased restlessness, aches, and pains are signs that you are progressing and practicing properly. They also indicate that your mind is more sensitive and aware. When you feel discomfort, smile. These uncomfortable sensations provide opportunity to develop equanimity. If you focus on your breathing and observe these sensations without reacting, you will be well on your way to greater mindmastery, self-control, and focus.

There is no mystery to why you feel agitated or uncomfortable; a lot is going on inside your body. You are a living organism with millions of cells busily multiplying, moving, colliding, and dying. More than 10,000 chemical reactions occur in your brain every second. Neurotransmitters, electrical impulses, biochemical reactions, hormones, and nerve signals are continually creating pleasant and unpleasant sensations throughout your body. Whether you are aware of them or not, you are consciously or unconsciously reacting to these sensations at all times, even when you are sleeping.

Whenever we experience pain, we try to make ourselves feel better. If we feel restless, we may fidget, mindlessly flip through a magazine, listen to music, or go shopping. If we feel sad or lonely, we might watch a movie, phone a friend, or eat comfort food. If our stomach or head hurts, we might take medicine or drink herbal tea. Some people use gambling, smoking, drugs, or alcohol to relieve pain, but these are dangerously addictive.

Another way to distract our attention away from pain is to escape into our imagination. Distracting ourselves certainly works for a while, but unfortunately does little to heal the root cause of our pain.

Life is full of difficulties, disappointments and crises. No person is immune to hardship, disease, and loss. Escaping life's inevitable pain through avoidance is not a long term, healthy solution. One of the best ways to weather life's storms is to develop equanimity. This means that no matter how bad you feel, no matter what conditions you must face, you will be able to keep a balanced mind.

Voluntary and Involuntary Attention

Habits form when we repeat behaviors without thinking. To change or stop an unhealthy habit, we must discover what underlying sensation is driving us to perform the behavior in the first place. For this self-investigation, we need to turn our attention within. Practicing breath awareness not only helps develop self-awareness, it teaches us how to be in the present moment. The other quality that we will need to prevent or stop bad habits is a trained voluntary attention—that part of the mind responsible for learning, focusing, and working toward goals.

Generally, we have two kinds of attention—voluntary and involuntary. Everyone, including animals is born with involuntary attention. It is the kind animals, babies, and small children have naturally without any special training. Involuntary attention is used throughout our lives to do things that require little effort or brainpower like walking, listening casually to music, mindlessly watching television, or surfing the Net. Involuntary attention enjoys randomly jumping around from one interesting or novel thing to the next. It likes to stay superficially busy and, as long as it stays busy, it's happy. Letting attention wander is enjoyable for the short term. Nevertheless, when life circumstances change and we want to educate ourselves, build lasting relationships, raise a family, and succeed in our career, involuntary attention is insufficient.

Voluntary attention, on the other hand, is the kind of attention developed through conscious repetition, mental work, and focused effort. Well-trained people like teachers, scientists, professors, surgeons, writers, artisans, and engineers have highly developed voluntary attentions.

If you are accustomed to only using involuntary attention, you will find doing breath awareness hard work. You may try a session or two, and then quit. Your habit of letting your attention jump from one thing to the next will make sitting and focusing difficult. Although feeling restless and distracted is not enjoyable, developing your attention is. A focused attention brings so many rewards; it is well worth the effort.

In this next sitting, try to recognize when a habit is controlling you. You may hear its voice complaining like a spoiled child saying, *I hate sitting still! I can't wait till this is over! I'm dying of boredom! I feel itchy all over.* Should you hear this complaining voice, smile, and go back to breath awareness. Your habit-mind may keep acting up, but every time it does, refocus on your breath. In this way, you develop your attention and you weaken your habit of restlessness.

Let us begin again. Start with a calm and peaceful mind. Remember to sit comfortably with your back and neck straight. Remove your glasses and rest your hands on your knees or in your lap. Remember to breathe through your nose, not your mouth. Close your eyes and fix your attention on your breath. We will sit for twenty minutes.

STUDENT PRACTICE SESSION (20 Minutes)

Two-minute Silent Practice
Feel the breath as it comes in through your nose. Feel the breath as it goes out. Observe your natural, normal, ordinary breath—as it is. If you are aware that your breathing is deep, acknowledge that your breathing is deep.

If you are aware that your breathing is quiet, acknowledge that your breathing is quiet. Sometimes air will pass through the right nostril; other times through the left nostril. Sometimes the air enters and leaves through both nostrils.

Five-minute Silent Practice
If you feel restless, bored, or any other physical discomfort simply acknowledge the unpleasant feeling, *Oh, I feel itchiness. I feel heat. I feel throbbing. I feel bored. I am restless.* Then go back to your breath.

Ten-minute Silent Practice

Feel the touch of every breath—as it comes in, as it goes out. Be aware of which nostril the breath is entering and leaving. If you are getting drowsy, straighten your back. If you wish to change your position, remember to do so slowly while staying focused on every breath.

Three-minute Silent Practice - Session Concludes

Good work. Open your eyes and make yourselves comfortable. You have all worked hard and it is time for a story.

THE LIGHTHOUSE KEEPER

Young Amy lived with her grandfather, the old Keeper of the Lighthouse. One day, he sadly announced, "Amy, you will have to take over my lighthouse duties." "But why, Grandfather?" she asked. Her grandfather explained, "I'm going blind. You are the only help I have. The stormy season is approaching and I will need you to light the kerosene lamp to prevent ships from crashing into the dangerous, rocky reef."

Amy was worried. Although she was only ten, she knew how important the lighthouse was. The reefs were dangerous. Unless ships could see them, they would crash. If she made a mistake, people on the ship might drown. "But Grandfather, I am too young," she nervously replied. He reassured her, "It's not your age that determines if you can do the job—it's your ability to stay focused and to pay attention. I know that you care for the safety of others. I am sure you will succeed. Tomorrow, I will begin teaching you how to operate the lighthouse properly."

For many nights Amy stood by, watching her grandfather in the lamp room. She learned how to ignite the kerosene lantern and how to adjust the lens to focus its rays of light. She learned how to direct the light toward the dangerous reef so it could be seen from afar. Her grandfather explained, "Sometimes, when there is a terrible storm, the wind will blow out the flame. You will have to stay awake all night. If the lamp goes out, you will have to ignite it immediately."

Grandfather's eyesight became worse; he could no longer see. A terrible storm was brewing. He called to Amy, "Go at once and light the lamp." Amy nervously climbed up the spiral stairs. At the top platform she fired up the lamp. She checked that everything was working. Then she sat on a chair watching the huge waves roll across the black sea. A furious wind howled and rain lashed against the windows. Waves pounded against the rocks below. Suddenly, far in the distance, there was a speck of light. Nervously she cried, "Oh no. A ship!"

Amy stared at the speck as it approached the deadly rocks. Time seemed to stop. The ship moved so slowly. It seemed like hours had passed. Amy's eyelids grew heavy. She nodded off. Suddenly, a wave crashed against the lighthouse. She woke up. Everything was dark. The lamp had gone out. Frantically, she scrambled to find matches. Soon, the lamp was burning again. She peered out the window at the black raging ocean. Where was it? Did the ship crash? She squinted hard. Finally, she saw a moving light. The ship was so close to the rocks. Amy cried, "Please don't crash. *Please.*" Frightened, she watched it maneuver past the deadly reef into the safety of the harbor. *Phew!*

Amy knew that she had made a huge mistake. For the rest of the night, she vowed to pay attention, "I will not fall asleep. I will keep the lamp burning. I will not let anyone die."

With strong determination, Amy stayed awake. Whenever the wind blew out the lamp, she immediately lit it again. When the sun broke through the clouds in the morning, she smiled. "I did it!"

She went to her grandfather and confessed, "I made a terrible mistake falling asleep last night. A ship almost crashed. People could have drowned." The old grandfather said, "Amy, you have learned the importance of paying attention. I would like to ask you to be the new Keeper of the Lighthouse. I know that sailors will be able to depend on you."

Just as Amy made a strong determination to stay alert and not to fall asleep, you are doing the same when focusing on your breath. The more determined you are, the stronger you become. You will become someone on whom others can depend; you will succeed at your goals.

Student Journal

Draw or write a story about your breath awareness experience today. Did you notice if any habits tried to overcome you while practicing? How did you deal with them? How can breath awareness help you in your daily life? How can it help in school or sports? How does a person change habits? You could also write a story from your imagination about something you have learned in Mindmastery.

CHECK-IN

- Could you feel the touch of breath on the small spot below your nose? How long did you focus on this point before you started thinking about something?

- Did you notice a tingling or vibrating sensation under your skin where your breath touches?

- Could you easily bring your focus back to the touch of breath?

- Did you have any experiences that were pleasant? Could you remain balanced? Did you notice any craving or aversion?

- Could you stay focused on your breath while changing your position? Could you stay focused when there were aches and pains in your body?

- Have you noticed if practicing breath awareness affects your relationships with people? Do you listen better? Do you empathize more?

Continuation of Practice Tip: For better digestion, weight control, and assimilation of food, become conscious of your eating habits. Conscious eating prevents us from eating out of blind response to underlying emotion. Eating often becomes a habit rather than a choice; these habits then control our choices. We may eat more than needed, for example, only because eating has become habit. We also may eat a particular food only because it satisfies a craving for a pleasant sensation. Cravings further compel us to eat too much or to eat unhealthy food.

STEP FOUR

Cultivating Wholesome Qualities

"Mindmastery helped me by making me learn how to focus on my thoughts and by telling me that I was the master of my mind. It helped me set more goals for myself and it helped me to be more considerate, and helped me to calm down!" —Ryan, Age 10

YOUR PRACTICE SESSION - STEP FOUR (50 Minutes)

Sit in a comfortable and relaxed position and commit to sitting the full fifty minutes. Do not move your body or open your eyes unless necessary. If you have to change your position, do so without interrupting your focus. Keep your entire attention focused on the subtle touch of breath at the entrance of your nose. If you feel discomfort elsewhere in your body, remember that pain is temporary and resume focusing only on breathing. When discomfort escalates, remind yourself that the goal of your practice is to develop equanimity.

When your mind is still, try to detect other sensations manifesting under the skin in the area around the entrance of your nostrils. You may feel itchiness, tickling, vibrating, throbbing, pulsating, heat, or stinging—every sensation is important. For a few minutes observe these sensations caused by bodily processes, cells moving, blood pumping, and nerves vibrating. After you are able to distinguish both kinds of sensations, return to only feeling the breath as it passes over the skin. Developing the ability to discriminate between the touch of breath on the skin's surface and the subtle sensations occurring directly below its surface indicates a sharp, well-trained attention.

During this longer sitting you might experience different physical and mental states ranging from relaxed and energized to sad and restless. Uncomfortable physical conditions indicate that suppressed negativity is manifesting as a feeling or sensation. When you become aware of discomfort or agitation, use the opportunity to develop equanimity. While experiencing discomfort, stay mindful of every breath. Should pain intensify, continue focusing only on your breath. If you become increasingly agitated, narrow your focus to a single point. When deep-rooted issues manifest they may overwhelm you with fear, doubt, depression, sadness, or resentment. Simply acknowledge whatever feeling is manifesting and then return to observing your breath. In this way, your attention will become particularly sharp and you will avoid fueling negativity with adverse reactions. Let nothing overpower your equanimity and peace. Be your own master! You may wish to review Check-in questions when you are finished.

TEACHER TIPS

One of the first things to do in the cultivation of attention is to learn to think of, and do, one thing at a time. Acquiring the "knack" or habit of attending closely to the thing that is before us, and then passing on to the next and treating it in the same way, is most conducive to success, and its practice is the best exercise for the cultivation of the faculty of attention.
—Paul Bruton, Quest of the Overself

Making Mindmastery Fun

It is important to keep breath awareness lessons enjoyable. If a child finds an experience unpleasant or tedious, there may be little incentive for him or her to continue practicing at home or even to attempt the exercise again later in life. To make sessions more fun, ensure that the sitting times are age appropriate, incorporate stories into the lessons, use humor, and provide time for journal writing, arts and crafts, and sharing.

The key to facilitating a meaningful and pleasurable experience is to ensure that students practice the technique properly. If they do, they will feel calm and energized, and will be motivated to continue. Most children like Mindmastery simply because they are with friends or others their age. Some also welcome the challenge and feel accomplished when they sit and focus for a prolonged stretch of time. Their memory of *I did it!* may give them the confidence to embrace other challenges in life. Other children love doing breath awareness because it connects them to that safe and peaceful place inside.

Try to keep the lessons relaxing by minimizing competition. Children often like to please their teacher or strive to be the best in the class. Remind children that breath awareness is not about who sits the longest, but how much equanimity is developed. For competitive students this may seem odd; for others, it comes as a relief.

Speak to the highest potential within each child and express confidence in his or her abilities. Express sincere interest in their progress by asking questions and listening to their explanations. Your encouraging words will water their wholesome seeds and latent strengths. Questions might include the following:

- Do you feel the touch of breath on your skin?
- Is it warm or cool, humid or dry?
- Do you keep your eyes closed for the whole session?
- Can you observe your discomfort before moving your position?
- When you move, can you stay focused on breathing?
- How many breaths can you stay with before losing focus?
- Do you have any questions about breath awareness?
- Do you understand what equanimity means?
- Why is equanimity important?

Feeling Breath, Nothing More

While practicing breath awareness, students might start counting or whispering words like *in, out*. They may talk about what they have been visualizing or imagining during breath awareness. Although these intellectual activities indicate that they do not quite understand how to do pure breath awareness, it does show that they are working seriously, making an effort to understand, and processing their experiences the best they can. Acknowledge their discoveries and then remind them to go back to their breath. Counting, verbalizing, and visualizing certainly help focus the mind quickly; however, focusing quickly is not the primary goal of breath awareness. When you notice a child resorting to these methods, acknowledge the benefits and then explain why adding words or visualizing pictures while practicing distracts the mind from actually *feeling* the breath.

You may discover that some children simply cannot feel the breath. Either their minds are preoccupied or they are confused about the technique. Explain that the breath can at times be very soft; even some adults do not feel it. Ask them to breathe harder until the cool, stinging air is felt inside the nose. Once felt, they can redirect their attention to the small area at the entrance of the nose, and try again. Going back and forth between these two areas is usually all that is needed. If a student still has trouble, have him or her breathe on the back of the hand and then refocus on feeling breath.

Some children may be still confused about what it means to *feel*. They might be imagining the breath as a light or stream flowing into the body. If you think that this happening, go through the above steps so they can experience the touch of breath. As soon as a child succeeds, he or she should resume normal breathing.

STUDENT INSTRUCTIONS - STEP FOUR

Cultivating Wholesome Qualities

Welcome to your fourth session of Mindmastery. Each one of you has worked seriously and may already feel more alert and attentive. Every time you practice breath awareness, even for just a few minutes, you are strengthening your attention muscle, sharpening your focus, and calming your restlessness.

For the past three sessions, you have been diligently training your excited, puppy-dog mind to sit still, pay attention, and obediently return to your breath when it wanders away. By repeatedly calling your attention back to your breath, your mind has become much stronger. A trained attention, like a well-trained dog, becomes a great friend that you can always depend on. A focused mind can help you accomplish everything you set out to do and the more you master your restless, wandering thoughts, the happier you will be.

We all want to live in a peaceful world that is free from war, racism, hatred, and greed. Although you might think that you are too young to make the world a better place, the contrary is true. Every time you practice breath awareness, you are making a difference. When you develop peacefulness inside yourself, you directly contribute to the peacefulness around you.

To help others, the first step is to heal our own mind of unhappy states like selfishness, greed, and anger. Before we can be of any help to anyone, we must transform unwholesome behaviors and negative mind states into helpful, healthy, and proactive ones. Otherwise no matter how noble our intentions, no matter how much we protest against wrongdoing, criticize people for the problems they are causing, or blame others for the unhappy conditions of our world, nothing will change. When we are peaceful and happy, everything we say or do will be rooted in peacefulness and our words and actions will contribute to the health and harmony of our world.

More often than not, it seems as if we have little control over our words and actions. Did you ever intend to be kind, but your words came out wrong and you hurt someone's feelings? Were you ever so mad that you thoughtlessly posted an insulting comment or photograph of someone on Facebook? Have you ever tried to control your anger, but lost your temper and shouted? Did you ever lose control and abuse someone? Have you ever promised to stop an unhealthy habit, but couldn't?

We think that we control what we do and say, but actually, we only have partial control. Despite what our conscious mind believes, our unconscious or subconscious mind controls much of our behavior. The subconscious is the part of our mind that we cannot see or control. Instincts, genetics, impulses, habits, conditioned behaviors, and forgotten dreams and memories make up the contents of our subconscious. If our subconscious is angry, fearful, or hateful, no matter how much we want to be a nice person, at some point these unhealthy states will overpower us and we may do something that harms others or ourselves.

For all our words and actions to be wholesome, both levels of mind— the conscious and subconscious—must be pure, loving, and peaceful. Although we do not have control over subconscious behaviors, we do have control over making our subconscious mind more peaceful and compassionate. When we heal the deeper level of mind and eradicate impurities like anger, greed, and selfishness, everything we do or say will be thoughtful, peaceful, and loving.

When we make a decision to do or say something, we are using our conscious mind—the part of the brain that we can mentally see, imagine, think about, and understand. The conscious mind knows, assesses, perceives, rationalizes, compares, learns, relates, reasons, loves, understands, and accepts. Because of all the intelligent and considerate things the conscious mind can do, we may think that it should be in control. However, the conscious mind has less control over our behavior than the subconscious. Even when we use self-control and will power, the subconscious can override our decisions. For example, our conscious mind clearly understands the risks of smoking cigarettes. Based on the information that we know, we make a decision to stop smoking. However, smoking has become an ingrained habit; no matter how hard we try to stop, we can't. This is because our subconscious has more control over conditioned and habitual behavior than our conscious mind.

To ensure that whatever you do or say is wholesome, you must clear your subconscious of unhealthy habits and harmful conditioning. This is difficult to do; after all how do you change something that you cannot see? Breath awareness can help with this. Breath awareness provides a way to "see" your subconscious. When you see or feel sensations caused by breath, you are actually connecting to your subconscious. Sensations and subconscious are always in communication with each another. Your subconscious is continually reacting to these sensations, even if you are unaware of what is going on. Therefore, by observing sensations, you are actually in touch with your deeper, hidden level of mind.

To illustrate these two levels of mind, compare your conscious and sub-conscious to a garden. The conscious mind is everything that you can see—the tangle of weeds, rocks, and soil. The subconscious mind is that part you cannot see—everything hidden beneath the surface, the buried rocks, worms, and dormant seeds. Now imagine that you are a gardener and your goal is to cultivate this unruly patch of garden and cultivate a bed of flowers. Before you begin your work, you assess what needs to be done. Your first job is to pull out the weeds. Once the surface is weed free, you can till the soil and plant your flower seeds.

Because you are an experienced gardener, you know that after you plant your seeds, weeds will still grow. That is because there are random seeds lying beneath the ground. Some seeds are desirable; others are not. In the first few weeks of tending your garden, you continuously uproot any new weeds. As well, when the tiny flowers start to grow, you care for them until they are established.

The hidden and buried seeds are like the contents of your subconscious mind. Ever since you were a young child, you have been planting seeds with words and actions. A kind deed, planted a kind seed. If you helped someone, spoke kindly, or exercised patience you will have planted helpful, kind, and patient seeds. Similarly, if you reacted with anger, you planted seeds of anger. An angry deed, planted an angry seed. Each one of us possesses both wholesome seeds like compassion and kind-ness, and harmful seeds like fear and doubt.

Doing breath awareness is a way to uproot unwanted seeds and weeds. When restlessness causes you to fidget or move around, refocus on your breath. This will calm your mind and restlessness has no option but to dissipate. When restlessness subsides, you feel calmer.

Even after your mind has calmed down, deep-rooted seeds will continue to surface. That is because you still have thousands of old seeds buried in your subconscious. Over and over again they will sprout and make you agitated, restless, bored, or frustrated. Nevertheless, your job remains the same. No matter what feelings manifest, you simply focus on your breath. By doing this continuously, you eventually clear your mind of all its buried negative seeds.

Once you are enjoying a more peaceful mind, you may want to know how to stop planting harmful seeds and how to keep planting healthy ones. How are these seeds buried in our subconscious in the first place? In your past, you may have performed a kind action and made someone happy. This event will be remembered as something positive. It becomes a healthy, happy memory; a healthy, happy seed. Similarly, if you perform a hurtful or careless action it too, will be stored, but this time as a negative, unhappy memory.

When you practice breath awareness, these forgotten memories may surface and manifest pleasant or unpleasant sensations. If you do not want to perpetuate your negative feelings, then you will have to exercise utmost calmness toward the unpleasantness that arises. The secret is to water only those surfacing states that you want to multiply. For instance, kindness and tolerance are two positive qualities. When you are kind and tolerant, you water these qualities in yourself. The same principle applies to negative states. When restlessness surfaces and you fidget and move around, you are actually watering your restlessness and making it worse. Instead, when restlessness surfaces and you water it with calmness, restlessness will diminish.

The secret to cultivating a beautiful mind is to first pull out unwanted weeds on the surface of the mind; plant wholesome seeds with calm and objective observation; refrain from planting unwholesome seeds with by being restless and reactive; and multiply your virtues by planting positive seeds by being peaceful and kind. In this way, your conscious and subconscious mind become pure and free of negative seeds. When this happens, everything you say or do will flow from a pure and peaceful mind.

In this next session, be aware of what seeds sprout. If you feel restless or agitated, know that states are manifesting. Calmly acknowledge what is happening and stay focused on your breath. Do not water the unwelcome seeds with more restlessness and agitation. Welcome these uncomfortable feelings with a smile, for they provide a wonderful opportunity to develop equanimity and cultivate your beautiful-mind garden. Let us begin. Sit comfortably keeping your back and neck straight. Fold your hands in your lap or place them on your knees. Close your eyes and begin focusing on your breath. We will be sitting for twenty-five minutes.

STUDENT PRACTICE SESSION (25 Minutes)

Five-minute Silent Practice
Breathe in and feel the breath. Breathe out and feel the breath. Feel it touch the skin below your nose. Does it feel warm? Is it cool? Is it a short breath? Is it a long breath? Is it deep? Is it quiet?

Observe your natural, normal breathing. Sometimes it will be rapid; other times slow. It makes no difference what kind of breath you are experiencing. Simply observe your breath as it is in the moment.

Is your breath passing in through your left nostril or your right nostril? Is it passing through both? Be like an alert doorkeeper at the entrance of your nose. When a breath enters, be aware. When the breath leaves, be aware. Your job is to watch each breath. Do not let a single breath pass through the entrance of your nostrils unnoticed.

If you cannot keep your eyes closed, look down at your hands. However, always keep your attention focused on the incoming and outgoing breath. Once you feel comfortable, close your eyes.

Five-minute Silent Practice
If you are restless, tired, or bored, acknowledge the discomfort and go back to your feeling your breath.

Ten-minute Silent Practice

If you get drowsy, take a few deep breaths. If you are still sleepy, stand up for a minute. When you stand up, continue feeling your breath. When you are more alert, sit again and resume your practice.

Five-minute Silent Practice - Session Concludes

Good! You may open your eyes. You have all worked hard weeding out your unwholesome seeds. You are becoming master gardeners cultivating qualities like patience, calmness, and focus. It is now time to relax and listen to a story.

SEEDS OF HAPPINESS

Every morning when Harold walked to his office, he passed Farmer Joe working in his flower garden. "Good morning, Joe!" he would call out. The old farmer would reply, "Good morning, Harold."

Harold enjoyed working at his office. He liked accounting and was good at adding and subtracting, keeping the company's books in order, and ensuring that bills were paid. However, over the years he started to feel that there was something missing in his life. When he was melancholy, he gazed out the window at Farmer Joe tending to his beautiful garden.

One day, walking home from work, he found a tiny, mysterious object on the pavement. *Could this be a seed?* He got home and phoned Farmer Joe. "Hello Joe, this is Harold speaking. I was wondering, how do you grow a seed?" Joe answered, "Well, it takes a little know-how, but it's easy. First, you press the seed into some earth, cover it with dirt, tap it gently, put it in a sunny location, and water it every second day. After that, all you do is wait until it sprouts."

Harold thanked Joe and immediately went to the store for supplies. He did exactly as Farmer Joe advised. He covered the seed with soil, kept the pot on a windowsill in the sunshine, and every second day he sprinkled it with water. Early each morning before he went to work, Harold longingly peered at the pot to see if the seed had sprouted. He dreamed about taking his beautiful flower to his office and imagined how happy he will be.

One morning—lo and behold—a pale green sprout pushed up through the soil. Harold was ecstatic! With each passing day his flower grew, and grew, and GREW. Harold knew that it was going to be the biggest flower ever. One morning, on his way to the office, Farmer Joe called out, "How's your plant?" Harold smiled proudly, "Thank-you, it's growing very well indeed."

A few weeks passed. Harold noticed something strange about his enormous plant. Its leaves were thorny; its stems were prickly. Its blossom, if you could call it a blossom, was a grey, scraggly tuft. Harold stared at the ugly flower—this wasn't a flower—this was a thorny bush!

Angry and disappointed, he phoned Farmer Joe, "You didn't tell me I was growing a miserable weed! I followed your instructions exactly. I paid close attention. I watered the seed every second day. And what do I get? An ugly old weed! *How could you do this to me?!!*" Farmer Joe calmly replied, "Well, what kind of seed did you plant?" "How am I supposed to know what kind of seed I planted?" cried Harold.

The farmer patiently explained, "Harold, you are describing what is generally known to be a "Thorny Bush". You must have planted a Thorny Bush seed. You cannot grow a flower from a thorny bush seed, no matter how much you want to. That's a law of nature, Harold. If you want a flower, plant a flower seed." Harold threw away his thorny bush. He had learned a lesson: If you want a beautiful flower, you have to plant beautiful flower seeds.

Harold's story also teaches us a lesson: If you plant ugly angry seeds with your words and actions, you will grow more anger. If you plant seeds of happiness with your kind words and helpful actions, you will grow happiness. Let us be wise gardeners and know that everything we do and say plants a seed in our minds. Ensure that you plant good, wholesome, and happy seeds and cultivate a beautiful mind-garden.

Student Journal

It is now time to express your own experiences. Begin by noting everything that you felt in today's session. Once you have written your list of observations, you can write your own story about cultivating your garden and planting seeds. Your story can be funny or serious. It could be something made up or something that happened to you. If you prefer to draw, that's great.

When you go to your journal stations, try not to step on anyone's cushion. Quietly proceed to your stations. We will work in silence for a few minutes so we can focus on our own experiences. If you need something, raise your hand.

After we finish, we can share our experiences, stories, drawings, and journal writings with each other. If you would like to read your own story to the group that would be great! Otherwise, if you would like me to read it aloud, I would be glad to do so.

CHECK-IN

- Could you narrow your focus to a small spot? Did you notice any vibrations and throbbing under the area of skin where the breath touches?

- Did you notice any changes in your state of mind from when you started sitting to when you finished? Did you have a few seconds of total concentration when your body felt as though it had no solidity or boundaries? Did you feel moments of joy?

- Did you notice that deeper issues started to surface when your mind became calm and quiet? Did these issues reveal themselves as thoughts? Memories? An imagined event? Or did you hear words and talking in your mind? After your mind became pre-occupied, could you refocus on your breath?

- Are you making healthier choices in your daily life? Are you more aware of your eating habits? Are you eating fewer pastries, sugar, and white flour? Are you choosing more natural, unprocessed food? Are you choosing to drink water over soft drinks? Do you have more energy for walking and exercising?

Continuation of Practice Tip: Breath awareness is not a diet program; however, what you eat will affect your ability to focus. If you consume food that irritates your system, causes your heart rate to accelerate, or dulls the mind, sitting still and concentrating will be that much more difficult.

Start reading the labels on food packages and make healthy choices. You are replenishing your cells, building muscles, and feeding your brain. Try to avoid food that contains white sugar, white flour, or devitalized ingredients.

STEP FIVE

Importance of Breath

"The first sitting was difficult for me today. My leg fell
asleep after about ten minutes. I was finding it hard to
focus. My mind kept wandering to a friend who just got
back from a trip and sent me a letter. It was interesting
to come to the realization that I had wandered off
and could come back to my breath." —Brett, Age 10

YOUR PRACTICE SESSION - STEP FIVE (60 Minutes)

One hour is an ideal length of time to practice breath awareness. Sitting for shorter sessions will calm the mind's surface and reduce agitation but may not allow deep transformation to take place. At first it might seem impossible to find an hour, but once you experience how much better your day unfolds and how problems diminish you will be motivated to practice for the longer period of time.

Start with a calm and peaceful mind. Put your worries aside for the hour. If you are stressed or preoccupied because you have to make plans or important decisions, remind yourself that you will be better equipped to do so after your practice. When the hour is over, revisit your concerns with a refreshed mind that is open to discovering creative solutions. No matter how serious the issues, sitting one hour guarantees more calmness, equanimity, and clarity.

Start by doing breath awareness for about thirty minutes by paying attention to the breath touching the area of skin at the entrance of your nose. Then, narrow your focus to a tiny point the size of a pinhead and continue feeling the breath on this spot. After a few minutes, try to detect a sensation on this spot. The sensation could be on the skin or just under the skin. It could be a pulsing, throbbing, stinging, tickling, or vibrating sensation. Stay with the sensation and note its changes; one minute it may sting; the next it may dissipate; the next it may tickle.

Observe the sensation as it is happening for as long as you can sustain attention. For about ten minutes watch how the sensation changes. It may disappear after a minute or two, but in its place another sensation will manifest. Often we become aware of a sensation and almost immediately become distracted and start thinking again. Staying with the changing sensation at the exact time it is occurring is difficult to do, but it is what the exercise requires. Once you have examined the sensation and noted its changes, resume focusing on your breath for the rest of the hour. When you have finished, consider the questions in *Check-in*.

TEACHER TIPS

*On life's journey, faith is nourishment, virtuous deeds are a shelter,
wisdom is the light by day, and right mindfulness is the protection
by night. If a man lives a pure life, nothing can destroy him.
If he has conquered greed, nothing can limit his freedom.*
—Attributed to Buddha

Why Focus on the Breath?

While teaching a group of children, check in on yourself from time to time to see if your mood or underlying stress is affecting them. It is not easy to be both the experienced, calm teacher, and the person responsible for running a program. Now and again, acknowledge your lack of focus, abrupt tone, or hasty movements, and whenever possible during the session practice breath awareness.

Be attentive to how the students are doing physically and emotionally. To help them relax, let them know they may move their positions if they are uncomfortable. Some children think they are not supposed to move, which causes stress. Children sometimes experience emotional upsurges while doing breath awareness; they may weep, make angry grimaces, tighten their lips, or start swaying back and forth. If you notice that someone is having difficulty you might address the group with a prompt to refocus on their breath. Remind them that emotions and feelings can be embraced and used to develop equanimity.

After sitting longer sessions, students may experience back pain, stiff shoulders, sweating, nausea, strain, numbness, tingling, or dizziness. If they write about these sensations in their journals or mention them to you, acknowledge the experience by asking specific questions about where the pain was, how intense it felt, and how long it lasted. Experiencing bodily sensations, separate from those caused by the breath, is an important stage. For some children, it is the first time they make a conscious connection to physical aches and pains without reacting to them. Encourage children to observe what is going on and to refrain from reacting, while using the opportunity to develop equanimity and focus. After a student acknowledges the other physical sensations, he or she should resume feeling the breath; children are not to spend too much time examining bodily sensations.

There are two reasons why children are not encouraged to focus on sensations other than those caused by the breath at the entrance of the nose. First, the goal of developing one-pointed focus could be compromised; attention grows stronger when it stays with one thing for an extended length of time. If attention were to jump from a sensation in the foot, to an ache in the back, and then jump to a throbbing in the head it would be counterproductive to developing one-pointed focus. Jumping from one sensation to another will not strengthen the attention "muscle" or sharpen focus. One of the primary goals for doing breath awareness is to develop one-pointed focus to help us perform introspective examinations. The second reason that children are not encouraged to focus on bodily sensations is that suppressed emotions can be triggered and brought to the surface. Unless you are an experienced meditation teacher, or trained to deal with psychological issues, it is best not to encourage children to work at this deeper level. If you notice students experiencing emotional turbulence, remind them to stay with their breath. If they continue to have problems, give them the option to do another activity—perhaps write, draw, or read.

Although examining sensations on other parts of the body is not an appropriate exercise for younger children, it is an excellent technique for adults. In *Your Practice* – Step Nine, you will be introduced to several other methods that can be used to observe bodily sensation. Although this book is limited to teaching breath awareness only, these other techniques can deepen your Truth experience. I highly recommend learning vipassana or insight meditation. Vipassana, is always taught together with breath awareness and provides an effective mind-purifying meditation, beneficial for dissolving unhealthy mental conditioning.

Why Focus on Natural Breath?
It is important for students to understand why breath is the object used to develop concentration. Some focus training and meditation techniques utilize symbols, pictures, statues, words, mantras, images, concepts, music, color, sounds, or visualization. Your students may ask why the breath awareness technique only uses one's breath. There are several reasons. The first reason is that breath is conveniently with you from the moment you are born and will be with you until the moment you die. Wherever you go, no matter what time of day, and no matter what you are doing, you can always direct your attention to your breath.

The second reason is that breath is part of your physical reality. It is neither imagined nor abstract, and if you want to know yourself you must start by examining and experiencing a part of you that is real.

The third reason is that breathing is both an automatic, involuntary body function, and a bodily process that we have temporary control over. Not all of our organs or physiological processes have this dual characteristic. The liver, for instance, is not something we can control. Breath can be observed either as it happens naturally, or as it is controlled. We can hold our breath, breathe deeply or lightly, direct breath into different parts of our lungs or stomach, and we can regulate how slowly or quickly we breathe. The exercise of observing our naturally occurring breath trains us to stop controlling and to start investigating ourselves objectively. This objectivity is a valuable skill.

The fourth reason why breath makes an excellent object to focus on is that it reflects your state of mind and lets you discover more about yourself. When your breathing is soft and rhythmic your mind state may be peaceful. When your breathing is short and irregular your mind may be afraid. When your breathing is hard and fast you may be angry.

The fifth reason to use only breath is that we can change, regulate, control, or manipulate our breathing to change our state of mind. For instance, when we are anxious, we can slow our breathing to diminish anxiety. As you can see, the mind influences our breathing and we can influence our mind with how we breathe.

The final and most important reason for choosing breath as our object of focus is that it provides a way to connect with the unconscious. Most of us believe that the unconscious and subconscious are inaccessible and remain forever hidden. However, this is not exactly so. When we perform breath awareness we gain access to the unconscious via the sensations that we consciously experience.

Sensations—A Bridge Between the Conscious and the Unconscious

Your unconscious mind is continually responding, communicating, and reacting to pleasant, painful, and neutral sensations. These sensations are caused by millions of physiological processes, hormone secretions, neurotransmitters, biochemistry, and molecular changes taking place inside your body. Even when you are asleep your unconscious mind is actively responding to these sensations.

Oftentimes, you are only semi-conscious of the subtle sensations that are continually being registered by your unconscious mind. When sensations intensify, however, like a headache or indigestion, you become aware of them. Breath awareness makes your attention so sharp that you become capable of feeling the subtlest sensation that would normally go unnoticed. The subtler the sensation, the more you experience what the unconscious mind feels. Because both your conscious and unconscious feel sensation, it is the common ground experienced by both levels of consciousness. Sensation, then, is a way to experience our deeper levels of mind.

We spend most of our lives reacting blindly to sensation. By repeatedly reacting to sensation, we form habits and conditioned behaviors. The more conscious we become of sensation, the more aware we become of our subsequent reaction to sensation, the more we experience and understand the root cause of our behavior and habits. We literally get in "touch" with the very impulses that control and govern our actions, reactions, and habits. Once we experience the sensations that trigger our impulsive behaviors, we have the opportunity to change our ingrained behavioral patterns.

By remaining calm and not reacting to either pleasant or unpleasant sensations as you normally would, you begin change and modify your unconscious behavioral responses. Once you feel a sensation, even one that is almost imperceptible, you have something tangible to work with. You can observe, feel, and experience the sensation, however painful or pleasurable, and refrain from reacting to it. By not reacting, you transform your conditioned response to the sensation at its source—the root of habits and instincts. Breath awareness provides a method to alter, modify, and transform ingrained conditioning, impulsive reactions, and instinctive behaviors.

Another phenomenon that occurs when you objectively observe a sensation is that you actually change the sensation by watching it. This change could be caused by the mental energy projected onto the sensation and may explain the theory of positive thinking. Once we change a sensation by observing it, our unconscious will naturally respond to it in a different way. For example, if we are feeling irritable but stay calm and observe our irritability, eventually the feeling changes and we feel peaceful. The unconscious mind then responds to the peaceful feeling and reacts accordingly. Breath awareness, then, can transform the way the unconscious mind reacts to sensations, and it can also transform sensations so they no longer trigger reactions.

STUDENT INSTRUCTIONS - STEP FIVE

Importance of Breath

Welcome to your fifth session of Mindmastery. You have all worked seriously and learned a great deal about your breath. Now would be a good time to clarify why we choose breath as our object of focus rather than something else like a picture, math equation, music, or the imagination.

There are several reasons why breath makes an excellent object to focus on. First, breath is with you from the moment you are born until the moment you die. You can practice breath awareness anytime, anywhere. You can practice in the shower or while watching a hockey game. You can practice while riding the bus or lying in bed. You can practice before an exam or a competition. You can even practice when someone is scolding you. No matter what situation you find yourself in, your breath will always be there, like your very best friend.

Another reason why breath makes a good object of focus is that it tells you about your state of mind. Can you remember what happened to your breath when you were afraid or scared? Did it stop? Did it become irregular and fast? What happened to your breath when you were upset or angry? Did it become louder? Did you hyperventilate? What is your breath doing right now and how does it reflect your present state of mind?

Because breath is both an automatic process and something controllable, it is good for training our attention. Usually we breathe without even thinking about it. Occasionally, we control our breathing by slowing it down, breathing deeply, or making it short and fast. When we practice breath awareness we try not to control our breath, rather we observe it as it naturally happens. Observing the breath as it happens, however, is not so easy to do. In the first few sessions you likely noticed that every time you directed your attention to your breath you either started breathing more deeply or had trouble breathing normally. Eventually you mastered the important skill of objective observation; like a scientist, you could examine your breath without interfering.

Observing natural breath is not easy, but because it is difficult to do it is valuable training. When we practice breath awareness, we develop the ability to observe reality as it naturally occurs without changing, manipulating, or controlling it. This is the way we learn who we are. The moment we stop *feeling* our breath is the moment we lose touch with our reality. We end up lost in imagination, which may be more amusing, but it does not awaken insight into who we are.

Six Reasons Why Breath is the Object of Focus

1. Breath is always with you.
2. By observing breath, you positively change your state of mind.
3. Focusing on breath trains you to observe objectively.
4. Experiencing breath is a way to experience your reality.
5. Breath is universal and can be used by everyone without conflicting with one's background, traditions, or beliefs.
6. Consciously feeling breath and its sensations connects you with your unconscious mind, and gives you a technique to change your conditioned responses and ingrained habits.

In our next session, pay close attention to your breath. Note how it affects your state of mind, thoughts, and emotions. Conversely, note how your state of mind, thoughts, and feelings affect your breathing. Remember, when you do breath awareness, do not control your breathing, simply observe it. Whenever you become distracted or lost in thought, acknowledge that you have lost touch with your present experience and bring your attention back to your breath.

Sit comfortably. Keep your back straight and your eyes closed. If you have to move to a more comfortable position, do so slowly and continue feeling your breath. We will sit for thirty minutes. Let us begin.

STUDENT PRACTICE SESSION (30 Minutes)

Five-minute Silent Practice

Feel the breath, your natural breath, your normal breath. Like a scientist, observe every breath as it is. Examine every detail of your breath. You are investigating the connection between your breath and your mind.

Ten-minute Silent Practice

If you are agitated or restless, narrow your focus to a tiny spot below your nose. If you feel pain, itchiness, or strain on any other part of your body, acknowledge the sensation and resume focusing on your breath.

Every time you return to your breath you are training your attention muscle. You are stopping your old habit of restlessness. Breathe in. Breathe out.

Ten-minute Silent Practice

If you are slouching, straighten your back. Stay alert. If you cannot feel the touch of breath, breathe harder. Once you feel the breath, go back to soft, normal, natural breathing. Examine every breath.

Acknowledge each breath. Is it a long breath? Is it a short breath? Is it warm? Is it cool? You are studying your breath but you are also studying your mind. By observing your breath, you are calming your mind.

Five-minute Silent Practice - Session Concludes

You may open your eyes. Before we continue, you may change your position. Remember to move slowly and considerately. Others around you will be happy that you are being considerate. Well done! It is time for a story.

TREASURE IN THE POND

Once upon a time there lived a wealthy king who had everything he wanted—enormous castles, stables of fine stallions, a lovely queen, a beautiful daughter, a thousand servants, an army, and more luxuries than you could imagine. Despite all his wealth, the king was always dissatisfied, agitated, angry, and miserable. No one could understand how such a wealthy king could be so unhappy. Well, except for one person.

The problem started years ago on the day of the king's royal coronation. The meek servant who was setting the jeweled crown on the king's head whispered in his ear, "Oh mighty King, you have more riches than anyone in the whole kingdom, however, may I offer my humble observation. Even if you possess all the riches in the world, there is one treasure you might never have." These words made the king terribly unhappy—he hated the idea of not getting everything he wanted.

Since the coronation, not a day passed without these unsettling words echoing in the king's mind. Whatever this mysterious thing was, he wanted it more than anything in the whole world! And until he got it, he would remain forever miserable. Unable to tolerate it any longer, he made a public announcement: *He who brings the king the ultimate treasure will inherit the entire kingdom.*

A few days later an old peasant requested to speak with the king. "O, honorable King, I know where the treasure lies." "You do?" shouted the king, "Then give it to me!" The peasant apologized, "I am sorry, I cannot give it to you. It is not for me to give." Infuriated, the king yelled, "Then, I demand you to tell me where it is!" The peasant calmly replied, "Majesty, it lies yonder in the courtyard pond."

The infuriated king stormed off to his royal pond ranting and raving the whole way there. He stopped at the water's edge and continued crying and cursing. His hot breath blew across the pond creating wild ripples and waves. Tears flooded his eyes making everything blurry. "So, where is this so-called treasure? I can't see a thing!" he cried. The peasant who had shown him the way, spoke kindly, "You cannot see the treasure if your eyes are full of tears or the water's surface is agitated. Stop shouting and cursing, crying and wailing and then you will see it. The king tried to calm down, but it was impossible. "May I humbly suggest, noble King, do breath awareness." "What are you asking me to do?!" shouted the king. The man patiently explained, "Feel your breath as it comes in. Then feel it as it goes out."

Reluctantly, the king breathed in and felt the cool touch of breath. Then he breathed out and felt the warm touch of breath. After a few minutes, his tears stopped flowing and his breathing was quiet. As he continued, his anger dissipated and his mind grew calm. Then something magical happened—the pond's agitated surface became smooth like a mirror. The king peered down at the water's crystal clear surface and saw his reflection. His face was tranquil, his eyes sparkled, and he was smiling. He had never seen himself like this before. His reflection awakened in him a feeling of peace and contentment. For the first time in his life, the king felt truly happy.

At once, he realized that he had found the treasure. He turned to the man who had led him to the pond. "Thank you for helping me find this treasure. It is indeed the most precious gift of all, and without you leading the way, I would never have discovered it. My kingdom is yours." The old peasant smiled, "Noble King, that won't be necessary. I have already received your gift—your happiness is my reward."

Student Journal

Here is a list of questions that will help children reflect on what they have been experiencing. Their answers will indicate how well they understand the technique and if they are having any problems. Once they have spent some time writing or drawing their observations, they may wish to create their own stories.

Student Journal Questions

- Could you feel the touch of breath?
- Could you narrow your focus to a small point?
- What temperature was your breath coming in and going out?
- How long could you sit without moving?
- When your mind wandered could you bring your focus back?
- Did you feel uncomfortable? Could you remain sitting still?
- Could you stay focused even when changing your position?
- Could you keep your eyes closed the whole time?
- Have you noticed any changes in yourself?
- Was your experience different from previous sessions?
- Have you felt a connection between your thoughts and feelings?
- Do you recognize any persistent habits or behaviors?
- Does your restlessness calm down after sitting?
- Can you explain how to practice breath awareness to someone?
- How does wholesome conduct help your ability to focus?
- Have you been able to use breath awareness in your daily life?

CHECK-IN

- Could you stay focused on one tiny point directly below your nose? Could you feel the tingling of the skin or vibration below the skin? Could you stay with the sensation for a while?

- Did the sensation change its characteristics? Could you stay with the beginning, middle, and end of each manifesting sensation?

- If you moved your position to get more comfortable, did you stay focused on your breath even while moving? Did you notice more aches and pains, or less? Could you remain focused and equanimous despite discomfort?

- Are you noticing small changes in how quickly or impulsively you respond to things that happen to you? Do you notice that there is a longer space between when you first perceive some-thing and when you react to it?

- Have you noticed a change in how quickly you can re-establish a calm mind despite waves of depression or unhappiness?

Continuation of Practice Tip: You may find yourself in an argument with another person when trying to prove your point or defend a belief. When you become aware of the escalation and that the conversation seems futile, direct your attention to your breath. While focusing on your breath, listen to what your partner, child, friend, or co-worker is saying. Even if what they are saying continues to frustrate you, there is no need to react blindly. Turn your attention inside your body and pin-point exactly where your body is feeling heat, tension, strain, or discom-fort. As you regain calmness, you might choose to ask sincere questions, but be aware that the responses you receive may again trigger more anger. Acknowledge your angry feeling and then refocus on your breath. If you can examine your reactions and their accompanying sen-sations, even while engaged in a heated discussion, you will prevent an emotional escalation. Your attentiveness and calm mind will prevent further miscommunication.

STEP SIX

Uprooting Negative Seeds

"I KEPT MY EYES CLOSED THE ABSOLUTE WHOLE
TIME! This is the first time I wasn't restless. I only moved
a couple times but that was because I hurt my ankle on
Tuesday. I am proud of myself today!" —Joel, Age 9

YOUR PRACTICE SESSION - STEP SIX (60 Minutes)

Doing breath awareness for one hour each day will make a significant difference in the way you feel and how you effect deep changes within yourself. To help you experience breath awareness at a profound level, your remaining sitting sessions will be for sixty minutes. Eventually, you may be inspired to sit twice a day and enjoy even greater inner transformation and peace.

As before, start your sitting with a calm and peaceful mind letting nothing disturb you. This is an important exercise, not just for you, but for the people you work and live with. They too benefit from your peace and happiness. Set your troubles aside and work diligently with the greatest determination. Ensure that your back remains erect, your chin is tucked in slightly, and that you breathe through your nose.

For the first twenty minutes narrow your focus to a small spot directly below your nose. Take note of the changing characteristics of your breath and the different sensations it creates on your skin. A narrow focus sharpens attention. When your mind is alert and focused, begin to examine the sensations on and under your skin at the entrance of your nose. Examine the changing characteristics of each sensation as it manifests, stays a while, and then dissipates.

There are no special or particular sensations to feel. All sensations have the same characteristics in that they arise, stay a while, diminish, and dissipate. All sensations are of equal importance. They will range in intensity from soft and pleasant to stinging and unpleasant. They may tickle, itch, sting, pulsate, throb, feel warm, or cool. For as long as you can, stay focused on one single sensation until it disappears. Then pay attention to the next sensation that takes its place. See if you can follow the sensation as it moves under or over the skin. Once you have observed sensation in this manner for a while, return to feeling your breath.

When your mind is still, forgotten memories rise up and become conscious. These memories may form thoughts, images, scenes, or voices and are usually accompanied by a feeling or emotion. When this happens, acknowledge what is happening and then resume feeling your breath. Within a minute or two, you may notice a sensation intensifying somewhere on your body. If it is unpleasant, you may feel your back or leg aching. If the sensation is pleasant, you may feel aroused, elated, inspired, or energized. Acknowledge the pleasant or unpleasant sensations, and resume focusing on breath.

These sensations may be the manifestation of a memory or mind state. No matter how they feel, whether pleasant or unpleasant, refrain from clinging, craving, resenting, or developing any kind of aversion or attachment toward them. Acknowledge that they have arisen and then continue paying attention to your breath. When discomfort, uneasiness, or emotions manifest into sensations on the body, it is a sign that the breath awareness technique is working. Your job always remains the same—to continue objectively observing your breath without reacting to whatever else you are experiencing.

If you remain focused on your breath, mind states such as restlessness, impatience, boredom, doubt, frustration, or annoyance may intensify and overwhelm you. This is another good sign indicating that your concentration is very deep. Welcome the unpleasant feelings and understand that they are providing you with an opportunity to transform old conditioning. Smile, stay calm, and develop your equanimity.

For the remaining minutes of your session, stay completely focused on your breathing without moving a muscle. Remaining focused will develop your willpower and transform your old habit of quitting when the going gets tough. Stay determined, keep your eyes closed, and continue focusing on the incoming and outgoing breath. At the end of your practice, before jumping up and carrying on with your busy day, spend a few minutes reflecting on what you have experienced. Enjoy your heightened awareness and calm state. You might feel peaceful and want to forgive those persons who have broken your trust or disappointed you in some way. You might spend a few moments forgiving yourself for being insensitive to someone or for hurting his or her feelings. If you have time, consider the questions in your *Check-in*.

TEACHER TIPS

...Grant me the serenity to accept the things I cannot change, the courage
to change the things I can, and the wisdom to know the difference.
—Reinhold Niebuhr

Cultivating Wholesome Qualities

By Step Six students will be comfortable with their sitting routine and familiar with practicing breath awareness. Having succeeded at sitting for longer periods, they may have learned more about themselves and also awakened valuable insight into how their minds work.

Gaining knowledge through experience—this is what the children are doing—is different from the academic learning provided in school. School education primarily involves intellectual work—reading, researching, and listening to others. It generally teaches secondhand, indirect, or *apparent* knowledge. Students listen to lectures, watch films, do research, memorize facts and theories, and spend time acquiring abstract concepts and learning about other people's ideas. This kind of knowledge is valuable and teaches us about society, politics, art, science, history, mathematics, literature, and communication. Despite education's usefulness, however, it lacks in areas such as strengthening mental faculties and awakening self-awareness.

Ironically, the original Latin meaning of the word *to educate,* coming from the word *educe,* had more to do with bringing out or developing the latent potential of a human through formal training. To educate meant to elicit or develop a person's own powers by strengthening their mental and physical faculties and cultivating character, morality, and wisdom.

Nowadays, the word *educate* seems to carry a different meaning. After twelve years of learning, there is no guarantee that the inner potential of a child has been either elicited or cultivated. We cannot be certain that a graduating teenager possesses a stronger mind and body than he or she did before starting school, not to mention having gained more self-awareness. It seems that many young people leave school with minimal skills, conditioned thinking, unhealthy bodies, and a lack of self-knowledge. Without criticizing the adequacy of our educational system, we should ask if it is doing its best to cultivate a child's potential. As a society, we should be concerned that a young person's mind be stronger, less conditioned, healthier, and more aware after years of classroom training. Education would then be fulfilling a worthy purpose and contributing to a better world. They say a learned man talks intelligently about many things, but the uneducated man who knows himself possesses real knowledge. Although many well-educated people know a great deal, they may not have the self-knowledge that leads to more happiness and health. There is nothing wrong with education provided it does not minimize a student's opportunity to achieve experiential knowledge.

Our Sensitive Mind Antenna

Practicing breath awareness makes the mind acutely sensitive and allows us to enjoy life more. A sharp, sensitive mind, like an antenna, can detect subtle vibrations like those of joy, aesthetic beauty, intuition, and love. Young children, whose minds are relatively unadulterated and sensitive, are by nature more joyous. However, as they are exposed to excessive sensory stimulation, lack of exercise, unhealthy diet and environment, and a lack of creativity, their minds tend to grow apathetic causing them to lose their optimism. Practicing breath awareness helps us to regain youthful elation.

A pure and cultivated mind enjoys immeasurable blissful states like awe when viewing a work of art, a sense of profound spirituality when listening to beautiful music, or inspiration when seeing a beautiful landscape or sunset, or feeling empathy and love for animals and people.

When the mind is concentrated, you or your students may experience your physical solidity dissolving into an energy field. You may no longer feel your legs, hands, or feet being separate "things". All body parts may feel merged into one delicate mass of vibrations. Sometimes this "dissolved" feeling happens when the mind has become fine-tuned and connected with the body's delicate and rapidly moving molecular or subatomic particles. Other times, it may occur after a prolonged stretch of one-pointed focus. Whatever the case, it is important to simply acknowledge the experience and then go back to feeling respiration.

The same instruction would apply to children. The experience may be unsettling for a child, and to prevent any fear or worry, advise the child to go back to feeling the breath. Reassure him or her, that this experience is perfectly natural, and will cause no physical or psychological harm. The dissolving experience may or may not occur. Many people, who have been practicing breath awareness for years, have not experienced this state. Whether you experience it or not, has little to do with how well the technique is working. However, when it does happen, it can awaken the realization that you are not as solid as you thought you were. The experience reveals another dimension of your reality—and discovering more about yourself is the goal of this technique.

Feeling our body dissolve may cause us to see ourselves, and the world around us, differently. We may realize that everything, including the entire universe, is impermanent, changing, and transient. It may erode our notion that we are fixed and concrete entities. We may feel less separation and feel more unity. This sense of oneness may blossom into feelings of compassion. There are many exquisite experiences that can occur when the mind is concentrated. We have indeed, a "higher" self, and cultivating our mind may cause it to access mind states that are beyond our limited intellect and reason. The following quote by the Greek philosopher, Plotinus, beautifully describes the "superior" mind that is capable of experiencing that other truth within us:

> You ask, how can we know the infinite? I answer, not by reason. It is the office of reason to distinguish and define. The infinite, therefore, cannot be ranked among its objects. You can only apprehend the infinite by a faculty superior to reason, by entering into a state in which you are your finite self no longer – in which the divine essence is communicated to you. This is ecstasy. It is the liberation of your mind from its finite consciousness. Like can only apprehend like; when you thus cease to be finite, you become one with infinite. In the reduction of your soul to its simplest self, its divine essence, you realize this union – this identity.

Although focused concentration may awaken valuable insights and pleasant sensations, there is no point in striving toward attaining this kind of experience. Striving itself, defeats the purpose of developing equanimity toward whatever sensation naturally arises from practicing breath awareness. Your experience, whatever it is, will be dependent on your mind's concentration, purity, and sensitivity. Whenever something is dependent on something else, it is a *conditioned* state. To prevent yourself from perpetuating more craving, acknowledge the feeling and then go back to your breath. Understand that all conditioned states, whether pleasant or unpleasant, have the same characteristic; they arise, stay a while, and then fade away. Ensure that you keep the goal of developing equanimity foremost in your mind, especially when guiding and instructing children in this technique.

Facilitating the Experience

You cannot teach children wisdom; but you can facilitate an experience that awakens insight into their own truth. Facilitating a meaningful experience is your primary responsibility when teaching children breath awareness. Providing explanations, elaborating on theories, or describing the different mind states might be more of a hindrance than a benefit. When students are given clear instructions on how to practice breath awareness properly, they come to experience and know everything there is to know by themselves.

Should you notice that a student has become preoccupied with mental imagery, concepts, counting, symbols, or visualization, remind them why we limit our object of focus to natural breath. As long as attention is focused on breathing, imagination will be less of a distraction. With that in mind, however, children often need to conceptualize in order to understand what they are doing. For some, breath awareness makes them think about their minds, thoughts, and feelings for the first time. In an effort to understand what is going on children might resort to symbols, comparisons, or mental illustrations that help them grasp what they are experiencing.

Some circumstances make it difficult for a person to perform breath awareness. Even though the mind can be as finely tuned as an antenna, it may lose its sensitivity and alertness when dulled by overstimulation and exposure to things like harsh music, garish colors, and violence in movies. An insensitive or "gross" mind will have difficulty feeling the subtle touch of breath. As well, breath awareness may be difficult to perform when a student is expecting or wanting something extraordinary to happen. The mind will be lost in the imagination. Some children might believe in magic and super powers as seen in movies and think that this is what they are going to achieve with breath awareness.

Such fantasies will distract a person from working properly. Watching ordinary, natural breath is a sobering experience full of physical unpleasantness, aches, pains, restlessness, fatigue, and boredom. Your job will be to enlighten students about why these experiences are important and what benefits can be realistically expected.

STUDENT INSTRUCTIONS - STEP SIX

Uprooting Negative Seeds

Welcome to your sixth session of Mindmastery. You have all worked very seriously and many of you can sit without moving your legs or opening your eyes for a whole session. Most of you are able to bring your attention back when it has wandered and to stay focused on breathing for several minutes at a time. These are signs that you are progressing, your attention is getting stronger, and that you are working properly.

We have discussed ways to cultivate our mind-gardens. We know that if we plant seeds of happiness, we grow happiness; we know if we plant angry seeds, we grow anger. We also understand that we have been planting seeds all our lives with our words and actions and have accumulated countless positive seeds as well as harmful ones.

We know that if we think negative, angry thoughts we water those deeply buried negative seeds of anger. And once anger begins to manifest in our conscious mind we become even angrier. If we continue fueling our anger, we continue rolling in anger. We have learned how to stop paying attention to negative thoughts and to stay focused on our breathing. We know that this is the way to break the cycle so we do not continue re-experiencing negative thoughts and feelings. When we stay focused on breath, we stop fueling the anger, and it becomes weak and eventually dissipates.

We also know that if we calmly and objectively observe our breath, our wholesome seeds are watered; seeds of kindness, patience, understanding, and love grow stronger. Some of you believe that you possess few positive seeds because you always feel impatient, angry, restless, lazy, or inconsiderate. Understand that we all have thousands of good seeds within us; they are just waiting for water. These are seeds of courage, kindness, empathy, compassion, patience, tolerance, generosity, and wisdom. The best way to grow these qualities is to water them with wholesome thoughts, words, and actions. Every time we perform a kind act, we water kindness within. Every time we have a loving thought, we water our compassion. Every time we do breath awareness we are watering our good qualities like equanimity, calmness, peace, patience, and love. Breath awareness cultivates these qualities, and the more we practice the more they will grow.

The secret to happiness is to clean out the buried negative seeds before they have a chance to sprout. If we fail to weed out anger, greed, and selfishness, they will one day sprout and cause us to feel bad, or to do something we will regret. We may lose our temper, hurt someone, get depressed, steal, or tell a lie.

Practicing breath awareness is an excellent way to rid the mind of its negative seeds. The job is simple to do, but takes strong determination. You will need sharp attention and a still mind because as long as your mind is distracted, negative seeds will stay buried. If you sit still and keep your attention fixed on the present moment—the touch of the incoming breath and the outgoing breath—you will allow the negative seeds to sprout. Once they manifest as a sensation or feeling, you will be able to deal with them using breath awareness.

How do you recognize when unwholesome seeds are surfacing? Well, if you have anger in you, you will start feeling angry or irritable. Your body will feel antsy and uncomfortable, your heart may start pounding, and your palms may start sweating. If restlessness manifests, you will feel restless and start squirming or fidgeting. If seeds of boredom start to sprout, you might fall asleep or get very drowsy.

Once you recognize that a negative state is manifesting, all you do is focus on your breath and not react. Not reacting means that you make a choice to observe objectively, rather than judging, criticizing, or resenting the unpleasant sensation. It means making a choice not to move, fidget, or allow your mind to get distracted. It means to act like a scientist who meticulously examines an unpleasant sensation and observes its characteristics—how it arises, stays a while, and then diminishes. In your next session, be determined to sit and observe whatever pleasant or unpleasant sensations or feelings manifest. To weed out negative states make a commitment not to react to manifesting sensations.

Angry or restless mind states cannot grow stronger if you stop giving them more angry or restless thoughts. If an angry man is burning up inside, what keeps his anger burning? Angry thoughts, angry words, and angry actions fuel his fire. However, if the angry man pours calm, peaceful thoughts on his inner fire, and pays no attention to his anger, his raging fire dies. The secret is to stay cool, calm, and collected while observing what is going on inside you. This is how you weed out negative seeds and plant healthier, happier seeds.

How to Transform Negative Mind States

- Sit quietly and focus on your incoming and outgoing breath.
- Allow suppressed mind states to surface.
- Acknowledge when a negative state, like restlessness, manifests.
- Recognize the unpleasant restlessness and choose not to react.
- Continue focusing on your breath.
- Observe how a sensation intensifies, stays a while, and then fades away.
- Note your mind becoming less restless.

Let us start again. Remember, observe whatever mind states manifest either as thoughts, feelings, or sensations, and without reacting to them, remain calmly focused on your incoming and outgoing breath. Use the next sitting session to weed your mind-garden of negative states and to cultivate positive qualities. We will practice breath awareness for thirty-five minutes.

STUDENT PRACTICE SESSION (35 Minutes)

Five-minute Silent Practice

Feel your breath, your natural, ordinary breath. Pay attention to every single breath. Sometimes it is warm; sometimes it is cool. Be mindful of which nostril the breath enters and which nostril it leaves.

Ten-minute Silent Practice

Breathe in. Breathe out. If you feel agitated, know that you are agitated and continue focusing on your breath. If you feel pain, itching, or throbbing, acknowledge that you feel uncomfortable sensations and then refocus on your breath.

If you feel sad, angry, bored, or frustrated, know that these are your negative mind states. Acknowledge them and continue focusing on your breath. Focusing is how you cultivate your mind-garden to be free of unhealthy conditioning.

Ten-minute Silent Practice
Breathe in. Breathe out. If you are slouching, straighten your back. Stay alert. If you cannot feel the touch of your breath, take a few hard breaths until you can, then resume normal breathing.

If your mind has wandered, acknowledge that it has wandered and bring it gently back to your breath. Keep your eyes closed and keep your hands folded in your lap or resting on your knees.

Ten-minute Silent Practice - Session Concludes
Excellent work. You have all practiced diligently and have learned how to observe what is happening to you without reacting to it. You are becoming wise gardeners, weeding out negative states and cultivating positive qualities of your mind. It is time for a story.

THE COWBOY AND HIS DONKEY

Once upon a time there lived a poor cowboy. All he owned was an old donkey. One day he was letting his donkey drink from a pond when a man rode up on a black stallion. "*Whoa!* Howdy Cowboy. Would you like to earn twenty pieces of gold?" "Twenty pieces of gold! That's a fortune!" exclaimed the cowboy and started thinking. *With so much money, I could buy a horse, 1,000 cattle, a grand mansion and would never have to work again.* Without any hesitation he asked, "How can I be of service, sir?" The stranger explained, "All you have to do is deliver this important package to the Sheriff in Gold Rush City."

The cowboy couldn't contain his excitement, "That's easy enough. I will leave immediately." The stranger grew serious and added, "There are two conditions that you must promise to fulfill. First, the package must arrive before sunrise. Second, under no circumstances whatsoever are you to open the package. Can you fulfill these conditions?" "Ya, absolutely sir! I will deliver the package before sunrise and will not open it. You have my word," he promised.

The cowboy tucked the precious parcel in his coat pocket, waved goodbye to the mysterious stranger, mounted his donkey, and commanded, "*Giddyup!*" But, his donkey did not budge. "I repeat, *Giddyup!*" Finally, his donkey started plodding along. The cowboy imagined the twenty pieces of gold. He pictured himself riding a powerful stallion while rounding up an impressive herd of cattle. Suddenly, he was jolted awake. His donkey had stopped. The cowboy looked around, "Where am I?" There was no road, just fields and rocks. "You inattentive donkey! Why did you wander off?" he complained. The cowboy pulled in the reins and steered his donkey around. One hour later they were back on the road heading toward Gold Rush City.

The sun began to set behind the hills. "Hurry, you slowpoke!" ordered the cowboy. The donkey poked along, one hoof at a time. The cowboy pictured himself sitting on the veranda of his grand mansion. A servant was pouring lemonade and a fiddler was serenading his sweetheart. Suddenly, a rock fell on his head. "Ouch!" Startled, the cowboy looked up wondering, *where am I?* He didn't recognize the cliffs that rose up steeply before him. "You ignorant, blind donkey! You should not have wandered off the road. I will never get the package to the Sheriff on time. I will lose the gold! I will remain forever poor." He yanked the reins and steered his donkey around. Two hours later, they were back on the road to Gold Rush City. Impatiently, the cowboy coaxed his donkey, "Move, you lazy mule. *Faster! Faster!*"

The donkey lumbered along as the sun went down. Evening grew dark so the cowboy lit a lantern and attached it to a stick. He held the stick ahead of the donkey to light up the road. While his donkey clumped along, the cowboy tried to guess what was in the mysterious package. *Certainly, it must be something far more valuable than twenty pieces of gold. Maybe diamonds? Maybe a treasure map? Maybe land titles?* The cowboy's mind ran wild with possibilities. The donkey stopped abruptly and the cowboy tumbled to the ground. The lantern smashed. "Ouch! You oblivious fool! Why did you stop?" "Ch-ch, ch-ch, Ch-ch." *Oh, no!* The cowboy recognized that dangerous rattling. He peered into the darkness and saw a snake. He scrambled back on his donkey. "Let's get out of here!" he hollered. Donkey toddled back to the road.

All night, the cowboy and his donkey moved forward at a snail's pace. With no light, it was hard to see anything. Again, the cowboy started thinking about the package. He became crazy with curiosity and greed. He started thinking to himself. *If I peeked inside, who would ever know? What harm could possibly come of it? I could take the diamonds and disappear. Everyone would believe that I drowned or got lost. I could get a new identity and make a life for myself in Canada.* Suddenly, he looked up. Dawn brightened the night sky. Ahead, he saw a familiar pond. *"What?"* he cried, "You dimwit donkey, you've gone the wrong way. We're right back where we started. Now I will never be rich! All because of you!" Filled with anger and regret, the cowboy ripped opened the package. He peered inside. Then he turned the package upside down and started shaking. Nothing? How could this be? The stranger on the stallion had played a trick on him. The cowboy stared at his donkey and realized who the real fool was. His failure was not because he did not reach Gold Rush City. His failure was not because he had opened the package. He failed because he had let his mind wander. Instead of staying alert and guiding his donkey, he absent-mindedly let him stray wherever it fancied.

With this realization, the cowboy made a promise to himself. *From this day on, I will stay alert, guide my distracted donkey-mind, and not ever wander off track again.* The cowboy hugged his donkey and apologized for blaming him for everything. Now, whenever the cowboy rides his donkey he stays alert, keeps the reins tight, and steers his donkey-mind toward his goals. This is how the cowboy got where he wanted to go and became rich in more ways than imaginable. After this lesson, the cowboy and his donkey traveled happily together reaching every destination they set out to achieve.

Student Journal

After you make notes about your experience in today's breath awareness session, write or illustrate your own story about what happens when we let our minds wander. You could also write a story about cultivating your mind-garden.

CHECK-IN

- Could you sit through the hour without changing positions? Could you stay focused on your breath despite uncomfortable sensations in your back, legs, head, or feet? Did pain or discomfort diminish when your mind became calmer? What states of mind did you experience? How did they change?

- Have you noticed any changes in your daily life and interactions with others? Does your calmness affect the people you are speaking to? Do you make healthier choices?

- In the past few days, have you observed how you react in heated debate or conversation? Are you listening more to other people without getting angry or opinionated?

- While sitting, did you experience how you fuel your anger with angry thoughts? Do you sometimes find yourself absorbed in or preoccupied with thoughts of anger or resentment? Are you using your breath to stay calm and to avoid an argument or prevent one from escalating?

Continuation of Practice Tip: When walking, running, dancing, exercising, or performing any kind of physical activity, try to stay connected with the sensations caused by your movements. Feel the wind on your legs, the sun on your shoulders, the sweat on your brow, the impact of the pavement under your feet. Become wholly immersed in the sensations of your present moment experience. The more you feel, the more you are living in the present.

STEP SEVEN

Developing Strong Determination

"I'm really happy that I joined. I think now that I have joined, it feels like I am a totally different person. Things don't bug me as much as they used to. I am trying to eat natural foods, and I find that I'm not as tired as I was." —Claire, Age 11

YOUR PRACTICE SESSION - STEP SEVEN (60 Minutes)

In this session you will be developing *strong determination*—a mental power that builds self-discipline, enables you to sit longer, eliminates restlessness, and develops one-pointed focus. Practicing strong determination establishes the kind of mental stillness needed to perform the penetrating examination of sensation. To execute strong determination, begin your sitting by making a conscious commitment to remain motionless for the hour and to sit through any discomfort that arises. Commit to keeping your eyes closed, your hands folded, your legs crossed, and your spine straight for the entire session.

Initially, you may worry that sitting this way could injure your body or aggravate an existing condition such as arthritis, back pain, or another physical ailment. When pain intensifies, try to remain motionless as best you can. Direct your attention toward the pain and observe its characteristics. Note where the pain is most intense and how it moves or changes. Note how it dissipates or weakens. If it becomes unbearable, move ever so slightly to relieve the pressure. Once you can bear the pain again, continue doing breath awareness.

To start this important session, assume a comfortable position and fix your attention on your incoming and outgoing breath. After a few minutes, narrow your attention to a smaller area. Feel only the touch of breath and do not let the sensations occurring under the skin distract you. If your mind wanders, acknowledge that it has wandered and resume focusing on your breath.

If you remain focused on a single spot for a length of time, you may begin to experience perfect concentration or *absorption*. Absorption feels as though your heavy, achy body has dissolved into pleasant vibrations. You may feel like a tiny speck suspended in infinite space, or like you are weightless as though some force is supporting you. This subtle energizing feeling can be pleasant and even blissful, possibly making you think you have arrived at the ultimate goal of breath awareness. However, as soon as you begin thinking these things, you have lost your focus. As well, the experience may change and the aches and pains may return.

When blissful sensations transition to not so blissful feelings, there is no need to feel disappointed or discouraged; you have neither lost anything nor have you regressed. As you progress along the path of developing strong determination, different concentration states will come and go. Remember your goal and remain balanced, knowing that change is inevitable. Understand that your body is merely a mass of vibrations and matter coexisting with consciousness and intelligence. Everything that you are, your thoughts, your feelings, your body, are in constant flux. Nothing is fixed; nothing is permanent. These realizations awaken insight into your true nature.

Practice perfect one-pointed concentration for about fifty minutes. For the remaining ten minutes, turn your attention inside your body and be mindful of everything that is happening. Feel the vibrating sensations in your scalp, head, face, eyes, neck, stomach, chest, arms, hands, torso, back, legs, feet, and toes. Be mindful of this whole-body experience; be aware of your reality as it is happening throughout your entire physical structure.

Sensation Awareness

Until now, you have been observing your physical reality as it manifests as sensation at the entrance of your nose. Limiting your examination to a small area quiets the mind and sharpens focus. Indeed, the aim of breath awareness is to develop laser-sharp focus that is capable of penetrating one's entire physical and mental structure on every level.

There are other sensation awareness techniques, such as *insight* and *vipassana* that use sensation as the object of focus. Vipassana, for example, expands the area of examination to include sensations felt both on the skin's surface and inside the body. These observation methods are fundamentally the same as breath awareness, only the area of examination encompasses the entire mind/body phenomenon. To perform a penetrating examination of internal sensations, a person requires both one-pointed focus and a wholesome foundation. All sensation awareness techniques, whether they examine a small area of the body or the entire mind and body share similar goals; namely, to calm and purify the mind, while awakening self-knowledge.

After your session ends, you might like to reflect on the questions in your *Check-in*.

TEACHER TIPS

*Afflictive emotions—our jealousy, anger, hatred, fear—can be put to
an end when you realize that these emotions are only temporary,
that they always pass on like clouds in the sky.* –Dalai Lama

Mindmastery is Non-competitive

By Step Seven, children will be competent in breath awareness and
might already notice changes in their behavior. Some may feel less restless, bored, or agitated. Others may have stopped habits such as fidgeting, eating junk food, or biting their nails. They may have better
concentration and feel more confident.

Depending on what students have experienced so far, the next session will be easy or difficult. If you think your group is ready to take on
a bigger challenge, it could be worthwhile to give students the choice to
exercise strong determination. Your job is to explain the benefits that
can come from the practice and to inspire students to embrace the challenge. If they have been working seriously through the six previous
lessons, they will likely want to move to this next stage.

Strong determination requires that students do breath awareness for
a set time without opening their eyes, moving their hands, or changing
their positions. Children who successfully sit still for this session will
remember the experience for the rest of their lives. Strong determination
not only develops endurance and willpower, it helps build a student's
self-confidence for other challenges in life.

Despite the good that can arise out of a session of strong determination, there are some cautionary notes. You should ensure that the practice does not incite competitiveness, as competition defeats the purpose
of learning for oneself. Competition disrupts the balance of mind and
can cause students to feel discouraged or disappointed. Competitiveness should be discouraged because practicing breath awareness is
never about how long one can sit, rather it is about gaining insight into
one's nature and developing equanimity toward whatever is happening.

When students practice a session of strong determination they will
focus exclusively on the breath, making a continuous effort not to miss a
single one. The exercise, like muscle training, causes the mind to be-

come laser sharp. With such a sharp observational tool, a student will be able to examine more precisely the breath and its sensations.

Exercising one's determination also disciplines the mind. And a disciplined mind can more easily control blind reactions and impulsive behavior by staying balanced, seeing clearly, and making good choices. Strong determination also develops one's ability to sit longer, which allows buried memories and negative mind states to manifest. Conversely, if the mind remains distracted and the body is restless, those memories and mind states stay hidden in the unconscious and cannot be transformed. An experienced student anticipates and welcomes the arrival of negative mind states, despite their unpleasantness, because they provide opportunity to develop equanimity.

Meeting the Challenge with a Healthy Attitude

Be aware that some students, often those you least expect, impose high expectations on themselves or feel pressure from their peers. For example, a student who suffers from ADHD may decide to challenge himself even more just to prove to others that he or she is capable. Be sensitive to each child's needs and discourage anything that will cause him or her to feel like a failure. Feeling disappointment will agitate the mind making breath awareness more difficult to perform.

Students might misinterpret your instructions to sit perfectly still as an imposed restriction. When instructing a session of strong determination, explain that it is a self-imposed challenge; if they choose to change positions they may do so. Most children are keen to meet this challenge. Once they experience the rewards they may be more willing to impose similar restrictions on themselves later in life, not with regret or resistance, rather with a knowing smile. Strong determination is a mental force and skill that can help a person accomplish personal goals.

STUDENT INSTRUCTIONS - STEP SEVEN

Developing Strong Determination

Welcome to your seventh Mindmastery session. You have all been working properly and have certainly experienced numerous benefits. You know how to calm your mind by focusing on your breath. You feel your mind becoming sharp—even a pin dropping to the floor makes you start. You know how to put thoughts in the background of your mind while remaining focused on your breath. Even when someone starts talking or there is a noise outside, you can stay with your breath. These are signs that you are developing strong focus.

You have also learned how to rid your mind of harmful seeds and how to cultivate wholesome qualities by remaining non-reactive despite uncomfortable sensation. Maybe your foot fell asleep and you chose simply to acknowledge that your foot fell asleep while you continued watching your breath. Maybe you felt an itch but made a choice not to scratch it. Perhaps an insect landed on your leg but you did nothing. These are signs that you are developing mastery over your reactive mind.

In this session, we will be learning how to practice *strong determination.* To do strong determination, you will commit to sitting absolutely still for the whole session. You will commit to not opening your eyes, fidgeting with your hands, or moving your legs. Previously when you were uncomfortable you shifted your position, but in this session you will make an effort not to move at all. Of course, this will be your choice. If you are having lots of discomfort do not feel forced to sit still; move slowly but keep your attention fixed on your breath.

To develop strong determination you will be exerting extra effort, which will greatly improve your concentration skills. Sometimes in life you have to perform difficult tasks—maybe climb a mountain, write an exam, control your anger, bear immense pain, or even save someone's life. When such events call for your help you will be more prepared having practiced strong determination in your daily sittings.

You probably already use strong determination in your life when you do sports, dance, or play an instrument. If you want to perform well, you make a strong commitment or promise to practice every day. Despite being tired, restless, or lacking confidence, you muster the energy and courage to practice. Later, when you accomplish your goal, you feel proud and happy.

To develop strong determination, we will sit for thirty-five minutes without moving. If it becomes too much for you, do not worry, just choose to change positions. If you feel disappointed in yourself, acknowledge the disappointing feeling and then go back to watching your breath. Remember that the real goal of breath awareness is to develop equanimity toward whatever pleasant or unpleasant feelings arise.

Let us practice strong determination. Make a commitment to yourself to sit for thirty-five minutes without moving. Your eyes will stay closed, your hands will remain folded in your lap, and your body will stay motionless. Sit comfortably keeping your back and neck straight. Tuck in your chin and relax your shoulders. Now focus your entire attention on the breath as it comes in, and as it goes out. Focus on the small area at the entrance of your nose without missing one single breath. We will sit for thirty-five minutes.

STUDENT PRACTICE SESSION (35 Minutes)

Ten-minute Silent Practice
Breathe in. Breathe out. Feel your natural, normal breath as it comes in, as it goes out. Examine every breath passing over the spot at the entrance of your nose.

Observe whatever is happening on this small area. Keep your eyes closed. Let nothing disturb your peace. Let none of your thoughts distract you from focusing.

Ten-minute Silent Practice
Breathe in. Breathe out. If you are agitated, know that agitation will pass. If you are restless, know that restlessness will pass. If you feel pain, know that pain is temporary and that it will arise, stay a while, and then eventually evaporate. If your mind has wandered, acknowledge that your mind has wandered. Resume focusing on your breath.

Do not let your wandering mind disturb your peace. Master your restless puppy dog mind. Train it to come back to your breath when it wanders away.

Ten-minute Silent Practice

Breathe in. Breathe out. If you are slouching, straighten your back. Stay alert. If you feel restless, narrow your focus to a tiny point. Do not miss a breath. Focusing will keep you awake and alert. You are in control of your mind. You are tranquil and balanced. Nothing can disturb you.

Five-minute Silent Practice - Session Concludes

Good. You have worked seriously. Even if you could only do strong determination for a few minutes, your focus and concentration will have improved. Your mind will be stronger. You may open your eyes. You have all developed strong determination. Let us relax and listen to a story.

THIS TOO WILL CHANGE

Once upon a time there was a world-renowned cyclist. He had won many races in his life, but was now very old. He called his grandsons to his bedside. "You boys have been good. When I die, I want to give you something. You will find a box in the garage marked, *For My Grandsons*." Later that night, the family gathered around the great cyclist, and said their final goodbyes.

The grandsons were sad, but also curious about the gift. They went to the garage and found a large crate. When they opened it, they saw two bicycles. One was a shiny silver, carbon fiber racing bike; the other was a heavy, rusty bike from the 1960's. The older grandson eyed the fancy bike and overwhelmed with greed he stated, "As I am the oldest grandson, surely Grandpa intended this newer bike for me." The younger brother accepted the old bike, grateful for his grandfather's gift.

The boys wanted to race like their grandfather and signed up for the upcoming Tour de Canada. The brothers started training feverishly. While they were out riding, the younger brother wondered about his old bike. Why did Grandpa treasure this bike? Why did he keep it all these years? One day, he noticed an inscription on its handlebars. The words read: *This too will change*. He repeated the words aloud, "This too will change." These words must mean something important. After all, his grandfather was one of the greatest cyclists in the world.

Whenever the two brothers were training, the older one would continually stop to show off his bike to onlookers. Whenever the older brother stopped, the younger brother kept on peddling. The older brother would then catch up and laugh at his rusty old bike. The younger brother trusted that his grandfather's bike was special and ignored his brother's ridiculing comments. The brothers would bike up steep hills. Despite having the lightweight bike, the older brother would start huffing, puffing, and complaining, "This hill is too steep! My legs hurt!" He would dismount and push his bike up the hill. The younger brother's legs burned too. However, he would reread the mysterious words: *This too will change*. Then he would grit his teeth, push the pedals as hard as he could, and ride to the summit. His burning muscles did not stop him from training. As always, the older brother would zoom past laughing, "Slow poke! With that clunky bike, you'll never win a race." The hurtful words made the younger brother sad, but then he remembered the words: *This too will change*. He ignored his brother's remarks and kept on training.

A month before the Tour, the brothers were speeding down a narrow road when a huge truck veered toward them. To avoid crashing, they sailed into a ditch. "Oh no!" shouted the older brother, "My bike is scratched!" He was so angry and upset he couldn't ride for days after the accident. The younger brother's bike was also damaged, but he repaired its bent wheel and continued training.

The big race day arrived. The two brothers waited at the starting line alongside a hundred international cyclists. *Ready. Set. Bang!* Off they flew. The older brother sped past everyone. He looked back at his brother and laughed, "I told you so!" Suddenly, he hit a curb and crashed. His younger brother crashed into him along with a pile of other racers. Angry and embarrassed, the older brother started to cry. His bike was totaled; its handlebars were twisted; and both wheels were crushed. He didn't even care that his brother's bike was also destroyed. A race official ran toward them carrying two new bikes, "Here guys use these." The older brother scowled and scoffed, "This bike is substandard." The younger brother accepted the modern, lightweight bike with a grateful smile and said, "Wow, thanks!" The two brothers mounted their new bikes and caught up with the other racers.

Then a miracle happened. When the younger brother started peddling, the bike shot forward at lightening speed. He rocketed past the other cyclists, and his brother. Seconds later, he broke away and was far ahead of the peloton. He could not understand why he was so incredibly fast. Then it dawned on him. The heavy bike had forced his legs to work harder and they became extra strong. His determination helped him peddle despite his burning muscles. He did not let hurtful remarks slow him down or stop him from training. With these inner strengths and a new bike, riding was much easier. He gritted his teeth, braved the pain, and with unwavering focus, he flew over the finish line!

In front of a cheering crowd, he humbly accepted a trophy and a $10,000 cash prize. His brother watched jealously. The younger brother felt happy receiving the prize; however, he remembered his grandfather's wise words. He smiled, knowing that the secret to real success is to accept that all things change. Sometimes life is hard. Sometimes it is easy. It is best to stay balanced with whatever hardships or happiness, ups or downs, or fame or fortune that life presents, and work steadily toward one's inner goals.

Student Journal

Students may go directly from sitting to doing art or writing. There is no need to offer any suggestions, ideas, themes, or questions. Just have their journal or art stations prepared, materials put out, and sit back and allow students to express whatever they wish. Children need encouragement and freedom to express the things that are important to them.

CHECK-IN

- Did you experience moments when you were absorbed in a concentrated mind state?

- Did you experience any natural phenomenon such as mental images, lights and colors, or internal sounds? Did you acknowledge the pleasant or interesting sensation, image, or sound and then refocus on the touch of breath?

- Did you notice any craving toward these interesting sensations?

- Were you aware of the vibrations arising, staying a while, then passing away in the small area of skin below your nose?

- Were you aware of how your thoughts and feelings kept changing?

- Were you aware of unconscious, suppressed issues rising up when your mind was still? Could you remain objective and balanced?

- Could you distinguish between the sensation caused by the touch of breath and the sensation caused by molecular movement and vibrations under the skin?

- Were you able to exercise strong determination for the hour and not open your eyes, hands, or change positions too frequently?

Continuation of Practice Tip: You can practice breath awareness with your eyes open wherever you are, whether in public, at a concert, riding the bus, or waiting for an appointment. If you have difficulty falling asleep at night, practice breath awareness for a few minutes. When concerns overwhelm you, acknowledge that you are fixating on your worries and fueling your negativity with more worrisome thoughts. After acknowledging what is happening, refocus on your breathing. If you would like to challenge yourself, and feel even more rewarded from your practice, begin sitting twice a day, one hour in the morning and one in the evening.

STEP EIGHT

Seven Stages of Mind Experience

"I think if I keep doing this for my whole life,
I would understand myself and be able to deal
with the outside world." —Sylvia, Age 14

YOUR PRACTICE SESSION - STEP EIGHT (60 minutes)

Sit comfortably. Start with a calm and still mind. Let nothing disturb your hour of sitting—no thoughts, no sounds, no discomfort, and no distractions. Breath awareness is the most important activity of your day. After you are finished sitting for one hour, all things in your life will unfold more smoothly. Decisions will come faster; thinking will be clearer; and emotions will be balanced. When your mind is equanimous, you will be equipped to deal with problems, plans, parenting, and work.

Begin focusing exclusively on the breath as it passes over the skin at the entrance of your nostrils. A penetrating examination of this limited area will awaken insights about your transient mind/body phenomenon. You will begin to experience the truth of impermanence—that all things are in constant flux and continually changing. You will soon realize, through experiencing this perpetual change, that there is nothing solid about you; nothing to cling to, nothing to crave, nothing to resent, and nothing to despise. This realization will make it clear that there is no point in reacting to your ever-changing reality, your intangible self.

In this session, when your mind wanders, observe where it has strayed. Take time to observe the thought, image, or mental words that have arisen in your mind. Is it a thought about what happened in the past? Is it a thought about what will happen in the future? Acknowledge that your mind has wandered into the past or the future. Then, examine the thought more precisely. Is it triggering a sensation? Is it causing you to feel emotional? Are these emotions or sensations triggering other thoughts? Have you become overwhelmed with regret or sadness? Do you feel angry or frustrated? Are you thinking about a disappointing incident? Again, take note of the thought and see if you can detect the sensation it is triggering.

Remember, every thought will manifest a physical sensation some-where on the body. Understand that your mind and its mental content and your bodily sensations are codependent and coexistent. One cannot exist without the other. Once you have acknowledged the mind/body, the thought/sensation connection, return to focusing on your breath.

After examining your thoughts and becoming aware of any sensations attached to these mental images and concepts, return to feeling respiration. After a few minutes of doing breath awareness, narrow your focus to the tiniest spot and feel the breath touching this spot. Narrowing your focus sharpens your attention and creates an ultrasensitive mind.

When your attention is thus focused, direct it away from the breath's touch and feel sensation below the skin's surface. You may feel a vibration or a stinging, pulsating, or a sense of warmth or coolness. Watch the sensation with penetrating focus and observe what transpires. Does the sensation intensify? Does it move around? Does it throb? Does it fade? When the sensation vanishes, fix your attention on the next sensation that arises in this area. Continue observing in the same manner until the hour is over. If you are restless and cannot narrow your focus, go back to feeling the touch of breath.

Maintain equanimity toward the various sensations. Remember that you are not seeking any extraordinary sensations; you are simply observing ordinary, natural sensations. Your attitude toward pleasant, neutral, or unpleasant sensations always remains equal—you have no preference. One sensation is no more or no less important. They are all just sensations—impermanent and changing. Acknowledge any striving toward a particular sensation or feeling. Acknowledge if you are seeking, yearning, or looking for something more pleasant or something less painful. Your task is simply to focus on either the touch of breath or on the sensation under the skin at the entrance of your nostrils.

In this session, you will have practiced switching your object of focus from the breath's touch on the skin to sensation under the skin. Examining and experiencing sensation is the essence of the breath awareness technique. Experiencing sensation is the key to experiencing your Truth. When your session is over, you may wish to reflect on the questions in *Check-in*.

TEACHER TIPS

The moment one gives close attention to anything, even a blade of grass, it becomes a mysterious, awesome, indescribable, magnificent world in itself. –Henry Miller

Voluntary and Involuntary Attention

Having completed seven sessions, you are now competent in practicing breath awareness. You may have increased your attention span and can stay with your breath several minutes at a time. You may also be able to narrow your area of focus to a tiny spot and feel the subtlest sensation.

Maybe you are gaining insight into how your mind works and how everything within your physical and mental structure is constantly changing. You are probably also experiencing how your calmness stays with you after your sitting and enhances your daily life, affecting your family and friends in a positive way.

Whatever your stage, now is a good time to pay attention and to examine closely the faculty of *attention*—the mental force or "muscle" responsible for "seeing" and "examining" vibrational and sensory input, and relaying this information to the cognitive departments of the brain.

The Faculty of Attention

In *Raja Yoga or Mental Development*, Dr. William Atkinson (Yogi Ramacharaka) explains attention and then goes on to stress the importance and value in developing this mental faculty. He writes, "The word attention is derived from two Latin words *ad tendere* meaning *to stretch toward* ... Attention means reaching the mind out to and focusing it upon something. The thought of an attentive person stretches out toward the object attended to, like a sharp wedge, the point of which is focused upon the object under consideration, the entire force of the thought being concentrated at that point." When you practice breath awareness, you are doing exactly what Atkinson describes—stretching your attention exclusively to the spot where breath touches the skin.

The attention, like a receptor, sponge, or antenna, naturally absorbs or picks up all internal and external information and vibrations that contact the senses, including the mind. You cannot shut off attention except perhaps when you are in an unconscious or dreamless state. As long as you are alive you have no choice but to absorb vibrations; vibrations are everywhere and are happening every moment of your life. Vibrations can be light, sound, sense, taste, smell, color, shape, feeling, or thought. Vibrations enter through one or more of your sense doors: light travels through the eyes, sound through the ears, touch through the skin, feelings through the nervous system, mental images and sounds through the mind, and so forth.

The secret to mind training is to know how to train the attention to be a useful, attentive tool, rather than letting it remain an indiscriminate receptor picking up anything that it comes into contact with. The attention can either unconsciously or semiconsciously receive whatever vibration enters the sense doors, or it can be proactive and conscious and pay attention to vibrations entering. A discerning mind will accurately perceive and "see" incoming vibrations, words, and images for what they are, and react or act accordingly.

Atkinson also observed that when vibrations make contact with one of our sense doors, our "I" (the will, ego, or that part of the brain that controls our actions) directs the attention to focus on the vibration. The attention obeys the I command and stretches toward the vibration of the object. For example, you see a blue painting at an art gallery and the I commands your eyes to look at it. The eyes pick up and receive the light and color vibrations. You may also notice varying shades of blue or delicate textures. The more you look, the more you notice. While your attention is studying, contemplating, relating, analyzing, and examining the blue color, your prolonged focus generates mental energy. As long as the I stays interested in the painting and keeps discovering new information, you are commanding your attention to stay focused on it. The longer the I stays connected with the artwork, the more mental energy will be generated.

Focused attention triggers one or more of the five senses (and the mind) to work harder: the eyes strain and squint trying to detect details, the ears perk up trying to hear the faintest of sounds, the nose breathes in slowly trying to detect nuances of odor, the fingertips touch with acute sensitivity trying to determine a material's texture. The energy that focused attention generates further energizes the I. The I, or ego, feels positively alert, engaged, and curious.

Once the *I* has gathered all the information it wants, it becomes disinterested in studying the object further and no longer needs to employ the attention. When the attention stops focusing, mind energy dissipates and thinking becomes scattered. This dissipated focus causes the *I* to feel a drop in energy, which the *I* perceives as unpleasant or boring. To rid itself of discomfort, the *I* immediately finds some other object to focus on and the cycle continues. The mind and the attention perpetually seek stimulation to keep engaged and active; when the mind is disengaged it feels lethargic and inactive.

The key to developing focus and generating mental interest is to prolong one's attention on an object, examining every detail or aspect of the thing and observing with a genuine motivation to learn. Initial feelings of disinterest, frustration, boredom, or apathy eventually transform into interest and curiosity. A person who is unaccustomed to enduring the mental strain associated with the initial stages of focusing often gives up before interest is sparked.

While observing an object or contemplating a concept, the attention can be applied to put the thing observed into focus, much like the lens of a camera. Once the object is sharp and clear, the mind starts to use its "higher" faculties to process the information. These faculties begin relating, judging, perceiving, reasoning, visualizing, memorizing, projecting, analyzing, deducing, and speculating. The mind processes all the incoming vibrations and makes note of the resulting experiences. The realizations formed from processing the information are then added to the mind's existing knowledge.

As well as psychological growth, the activity of paying attention also causes physiological changes in brain structure. Gray matter thickens, neural networks expand, connectivity between synapses increase, various mental faculties are activated, brain structures become more integrated, and intelligence deepens. Just as a muscle depletes blood, energy, and cellular tissue when exerted, the attention, when exerted, causes the mind to use up nutrients, energy, blood, and building materials. The body and brain quickly replenish and repair what has been depleted sending the attention faculty a slight excess of nutrients, blood, energy, and cells. This excess rebuilds a stronger faculty of attention.

The Importance of Clarity

Everything we see, imagine, think, hear, and feel, whether the information comes from our imagination or from the world around us, will first pass through the lens of our attention; therefore, the clearer the lens, the more accurate the picture. If the lens is out of focus or marred, the incoming vibrations will be vague or scattered. If incoming vibrations are fuzzy they cannot make a deep impression on the brain. Weak impressions cannot generate energy, which results in loss of interest.

When your phone signal breaks up and it becomes impossible to understand the garble you probably hang up. Similarly, if the mind receives distorted information, the mind gets misinformed and causes havoc. For example, if you hear your partner say something that you believe to be hurtful you may start reacting. Had you heard and understood the words clearly, however, you may have perceived no reason to react.

Attention is so necessary to understanding, that without some degree of it, ideas and perceptions that pass through the mind seem to disappear. One's ability to attend, more than any other skill, will facilitate a person's learning and comprehension. Some people say that genius is not created through education, but rather through a person's power of concentrated attention. One of the most important intellectual habits a person can acquire is the habit of attending exclusively to the matter at hand.

We all have the habit of letting our attention be what it naturally is— passive. We relax and let our attention receive whatever comes into its vicinity. We let our minds jump from one amusing thing to the next, and enjoy doing so. There is pleasure derived from letting the mind simply be stimulated by whatever novel thing is passing through. We could describe this as mindless fun. Children are especially vulnerable to candy-coated, titillating distractions—and the movie companies, junk food producers, and computer games exploit their vulnerability.

To counteract the unhealthy consequences that come from keeping the mind weak, inattentive, and continually distracted, parents and teachers can encourage children to do one thing at a time or to study one object exclusively. Drawing is an excellent exercise for developing one-pointed prolonged focus. Breath awareness, of course, is another method. There are many ways to help children train their naturally passive attention into being a useful tool. If you succeed at encouraging a child to study one object or subject for a prolonged stretch, the child's interest and mental energy will grow and inspire more curiosity. In this way, learning and mind development become enjoyable.

Involuntary and Voluntary Attention

Atkinson describes the two types or degrees of attention and states as follows:

> The first is the Attention directed within the mind upon mental objects and concepts. The other is the Attention directed outward upon objects external to ourselves. Likewise there may be drawn another distinction and division of attention into two classes, i.e. Attention attracted by some impression coming into consciousness without any conscious effort of the Will—this is called *Involuntary Attention*, for the Attention and Interest is caught by the attractiveness or novelty of the object. Attention directed to some object by an effort of the Will, is called *Voluntary Attention*. Involuntary Attention is quite common, and requires no special training. It is the most natural kind found in animals, small children, and sometimes the elderly. On the other hand, Voluntary Attention requires effort, will, and determination—a certain mental training (*Raga Yoga or Mental Development*, pg. 101, Yogi Publication Society).

Understanding attention and the importance of strengthening it will help you choose activities that promote mind development. As well, the understanding will allow you to choose activities that use involuntary attention like sun tanning, perusing a magazine, watching television, daydreaming, listening to music, or walking. Balancing the two kinds of activities is healthiest. Having enjoyed leisurely activities, for example, you might engage in activities like breath awareness, drawing, practicing an instrument, working, studying, writing, problem solving, or doing anything that requires focused attention.

There is nothing bad or unhealthy about letting the mind relax and be passively receptive to receiving stimulation and information from either our internal world or the world around us. Letting the attention wander in a less focused and goal directed way is essential to emotional, creative, and spiritual well-being. Doing so not only promotes divergent thinking, but also can cultivate the imagination and intuition. Children do better in academic work when they can balance intense focusing subjects like mathematics and science with relaxing activities like art, music, and sports. We all need time to contemplate, daydream, unwind, and give the mind opportunity to encounter new stimuli and ideas. The key is to balance relaxing, non-focused mental activity with attention training that builds mental stamina, attention, focus, and brainpower.

Generating Mental Energy

As discussed, our involuntary attention is active all the time and re-quires no real training. When a thing passes by one of the senses, the new or stimulating object comes into the *I* consciousness. The object might be shiny, quaint, colorful, exciting, sensational, or odd. The *I* commands the attention toward it; however, as soon as the stimulating object either loses its flavor or moves out of sight, the *I* loses interest. Soon, the *I* directs the involuntary attention to the next novel or stimu-lating item that comes into view. Similarly, when we flip through televi-sion channels, we engage our involuntary attention by spending only a minute or two on a program before becoming disinterested and chang-ing to the next channel. After flipping through channels we become increasingly frustrated, bored, and our minds become fatigued.

We are all familiar with surfing the Web, playing computer games, watching television, text messaging, jumping from one thing to the next, or multi-tasking. These pleasurable and exciting, yet short lived, activi-ties are what the involuntary attention enjoys most. A person who has the habit of letting his or her attention jump around will find it difficult to accomplish a challenging activity, study a subject thoroughly, per-form complicated tasks, or even stick to a healthy diet.

For completing tasks that are more arduous, trained attention is re-quired. This only happens through concentrated effort, will, repetitive training, perseverance, determination, endurance, practice, and focus. If your attention is trained you will find it easier to learn new things and to deepen your knowledge. You will possess a greater ability to think, contemplate, imagine, construct, perceive, relate, examine, judge, re-member, and comprehend.

Common obstacles that prevent children from developing attention include television, the Internet, electronic devices, iPods, and a lack of focused activities. Many of us wonder how fun activities such as these can be mind weakening when they give so much pleasure. The main problem lies in the amount of time spent engaged in these activities. Realistically, thousands of hours during a child's developmental years are required to develop voluntary attention. These hours are simply not available to children who are preoccupied with using their involuntary attention. What we are now seeing in society, in children and adults, is a massive attention deficit. When persons with attention deficit face situations that require stamina, tenacity, equanimity, focus, or endurance, they may not be able to do the task required because they simply do not possess sufficient mental power. Their incompetence may then lead them to feel hopeless, unintelligent, or insecure. In turn, these self-defeating emotions may cause a person to resort to even more distractions.

Awakening Interest and Curiosity

When people hear about breath awareness, many imagine that it must be boring and tedious. They may even start to yawn when you begin explaining how to do it, and show little interest in your newly discovered insights into the mind. Few people have actually paid any attention to the breath—that ordinary, uninteresting thing. Nevertheless, those who diligently study breath eventually experience how it becomes an interesting and meaningful object to focus on.

For the past seven *Your Practice* sessions you have been tirelessly paying attention to the breath. You know every detail about your breath—its delicate touch, its warmth or coolness, its tingling, and its itchiness in your nose. You have noticed that when your breath changes, so does your state of mind. You know that there is a beginning, a middle, and an end to every inhalation, and the same for every exhalation. You know when your breath is long, short, deep, hard, or shallow. Through examining all these characteristics of breath your attention has grown sharp and penetrating and your mind has become energized.

Whether a child is doing breath awareness or any other activity, when boredom sets in, it is because the child is not paying sufficient attention to the object or subject at hand. That subject could be a lecture, a book, an assignment, learning a new skill, or the breath. Boredom indicates a disengaged mind. As well, children who are given an object or subject to examine that they perceive as silly, insignificant, or irrelevant to their lives may quickly become disinterested or reject the task entirely.

Because of their natural tendency to lose interest, there are two main points to consider when helping children develop attention. One, children need to focus on something relevant to them. Two, they need to focus long enough to generate mental energy. These two factors are addressed when children practice breath awareness. First, studying breath is relevant. Studying one's self, one's mind, and one's body, are all subjects of great interest. Self-interest is a natural tendency even in children. What subject could be more relevant to a child's life than their mind, body, feelings, and breath? Second, observing breath for prolonged periods will generate interest and mental energy. This feels good and motivates children to exert greater effort. The experience reveals how inattentiveness and disinterest zap energy, while focusing generates energy.

Most children embrace breath awareness; they intuitively feel its relevance and power. The more they pay attention to their ordinary, "boring" breath, the more they experience a growing interest in their psychology and physiology. This experience teaches a valuable lesson— the more attention applied; the more interest generated. Once this phenomenon is understood, children can use focus to spark interest in any subject, whether that subject is interesting or not.

I Need My Music
If you have ever taught children or helped them with their homework, you may have heard them say, *I can't work without my music*. Many children use music to generate mental energy and stimulate the production of endorphins. As discussed, without sufficient mental power, most intellectual and physical tasks are burdensome or boring.

To compensate their lack of mental energy, many children resort to listening to music while doing academic or challenging tasks. Music keeps their minds stimulated so the work feels less tedious. There have been many studies proving the positive effects that certain music has on the brain, like enhancing concentration, improving memory, and relieving anxiety.

Listening to music can be an attention-developing activity, but generally, many young people use it as a stimulating background sound. Music engages a child's involuntary attention and is wonderfully relaxing. It can act as a background stimulus that causes the mind to feel more energetic. Unfortunately, when the background stimulus is removed, a child's mind may feel too lazy or bored to accomplish a laborious task like homework. Although a child might complete his or her work while listening to music, the attention muscle may not have been sufficiently exercised, and the mind's faculties may remain as weak as they were prior to doing the homework. Music, despite its energizing and relaxing attributes, can become a substitute or crutch for one's natural mental energy.

Sometimes Mindmastery students ask if they can listen to music while doing breath awareness, claiming it is more relaxing. Now, however, you can understand better why music is not used with this technique. It may be more difficult to concentrate on breathing without the aid of music, but the attention grows stronger by doing so.

STUDENT INSTRUCTIONS - STEP EIGHT

Seven Stages of Mind Experience

Welcome to your eighth session of Mindmastery. We only have a few more sessions to work seriously. Every minute that you focus on your breath, your mind becomes stronger. Breath awareness is like doing push-ups or jogging. Every time you practice, you strengthen your attention muscle. The stronger your mind becomes, the more chance you have at accomplishing goals and living a healthy and happy life.

Our goal is to become the masters of our restless, distracted minds. If we were to become masters of our minds, it would make sense to understand exactly what the mind is and what we are mastering. Now that you have sharpened your attention and calmed your restlessness, you are ready to more deeply exam this thing called mind.

Let us begin our examination by seeing what happens when the mind is exposed to the world around us, or the world within us. The following are some of the stages the mind goes through:

1) Mind Becomes Conscious of Something

We know that the mind is connected to our sense organs, namely our eyes, nose, ears, mouth, skin, and internal nervous system. Let us examine what happens when we see, hear, smell, taste, touch, and think. Take note of what is happening right now. Do you hear my words? Yes, your ears are picking up sound vibrations and these vibrations are connected to your mind. Do you see things in the room? Yes, your eyes are picking up light and color vibrations and sending these signals to your brain. Do you feel a sensation of warmth or coolness? Yes, your skin is picking up vibrations of temperature and sending signals to your brain.

Now, direct your attention inside yourself. Do you feel movement, throbbing, pain, or temperature? Yes, your internal nervous system is feeling vibrations and sending them to your brain. Do you hear a voice in your head or see images in your mind? Yes, imagined sounds and images are vibrations that send messages to your brain.

When your mind takes note of any vibration, whether coming from the external world or coming from your internal world, it receives a signal. When your mind receives a signal, it becomes conscious of it. When you feel the touch of breath on skin, you become conscious of the touch. When you see something, you become conscious of what you are seeing. Only when your mind becomes conscious of the vibration, do you become aware. If the mind does not notice, it is unaware.

2) Mind Perceives Sound, Light, and Sense Vibrations

After the mind perceives a vibration and becomes conscious, the next stage is to make sense of it. Your ears hear a sound, but does your mind know what the sound means? If you hear a foreign language, you hear sound vibrations but you may not know what the words mean. If you see an object, you may not recognize the object.

We have talked about conditioning. Conditioning plays an important role in how our minds understand and perceive vibrations. If we speak English, our minds have been conditioned to understand English words. When our ears pick up these sounds, we can make sense of what is being said. If we have been conditioned to recognize a black widow, when we see the shape and color of this spider, our conditioning will warn us that the insect is dangerous.

How we perceive the world is often based on how our minds have been conditioned. If our thinking has been influenced or shaped to believe that the death penalty or slavery is acceptable, then we will have no objection to them. If we have been conditioned to think that women should have no rights, we would accept this as normal. If we have been made to believe that our religion is the only religion, we would condemn others for their beliefs. Although conditioning is essential to understanding, it can be detrimental and destructive. Our responsibility lies in discerning between helpful behaviors and customs, and harmful beliefs and conditioning. Our duty lies in understanding how we have been shaped, and then how to free ourselves of harmful conditioning.

3) Mind Recognizes the Vibrations

Once the mind recognizes a light, sound, taste, or touch vibration, the attention has to go to its memory library to try and identify it. The process begins by assessing the vibration's shape, color, size, speed, tone, or whatever characteristics reveal themselves. The mind first looks for something that is familiar or recognizable. Is it a word? Is it a tree? Is it a shadow of a person? Is it a cloud? Is it music? Is it an animal? Is it a car? With lightning speed, the mind relies on its memory, intellect, reasoning ability, comprehension, and instinct to identify a vibration. Once the mind knows the object, situation, subject, concept, or thought, it attaches a name to it. Its name could be wolf, tree, coin, person, snake, theory, belief, song, or painting.

4) Mind Passes Judgment

The fourth stage is the most critical for changing habitual responses and conditioning. After perceiving vibrations and sensory input and determining what they are, the mind decides whether the sounds, shapes, or things are helpful, pleasing, harmful, or dangerous. How the mind judges will depend again on conditioning. For example, if an approaching person is recognized as an enemy, the mind will judge the situation as dangerous.

The mind begins by asking itself questions. Is this shape a person? Is he or she friendly or hostile? I hear music. Is it soothing or irritating? I hear someone speaking an opinion about me. Are the words insulting or complimentary? This is a painting. Is it depressing or uplifting? My teacher is speaking. Is the subject boring or interesting? This is a radio. Is it junk or rare antique? This is a woman. Is she attractive or unappealing? You will know that your mind is passing judgment when you hear your inner voice say things like, *This is good. I hate this. I love this person. This is awful. This makes me sad. This feels dangerous. This is beautiful. She is ugly. This is awful. He is great. This is friendly. This is nasty. This dog is dangerous.*

5) Mind Triggers the Production of Biochemistry

The fifth stage is a biochemical reaction within your body in response to what your mind has perceived and judged. Once your mind has passed judgment, it triggers a corresponding physiological and biochemical reaction flooding your body with chemicals that cause you to feel sensation. You might feel stressed, depressed, excited, infatuated, elated, fearful, or blissful. These feelings and emotions are rooted in sensations caused by the flood of biochemical processes felt by your mind.

Within milliseconds of the mind deciding whether a person, object, animal, word, taste, smell, or situation is friendly or hostile, the brain triggers the production of chemicals. These secretions assist a person in responding to the situation. They can suppress pain, induce pleasure, numb nerves, communicate signals to the brain and muscles, prepare the body to fight, or give a boost of energy for the person to run. There are hundreds of body and brain chemicals, neurotransmitters, and hormones such as dopamine, serotonin, adrenaline, and cortisol. These secretions fill the bloodstream, interact with other physical processes, and aid communication between cells and synapses.

If you hear your mind saying, *I like this,* it is because hormones such as endorphins, adrenaline, or dopamine are causing you to feel good. Without the presence of feel-good hormones you would not say that you *like* something. Alternatively, if the brain chemicals flooding your body cause irritability, fear, or stress you would say, *I hate this.* You can only hate, when you feel hate flooding your body and mind. On a superficial level, relationships thrive if the biochemistry between two people is pleasurable.

Sometimes the mind misjudges and reacts prematurely. It sees a shape, believes the thing is dangerous, and immediately produces fight or flight hormones such as adrenaline and noradrenaline. Later, when the mind recognizes the feared object for what it actually is, the rational mind realizes that it had needlessly overreacted. For example, if you see a snake on the road your mind triggers the production of adrenaline. This hormone accelerates your heart, dilates air passages, constricts blood vessels, and makes your face and palms sweat. Upon closer examination, however, you discover that it is not a snake but a piece of rope. The mind then stops producing adrenaline and you feel calm again.

As you can see, correct perception of a thing or situation will minimize unjustified brain chemical responses. When practicing breath awareness, we develop the ability to observe objectively, thereby preventing the production of inappropriate brain chemicals, which in turn cause us to react.

6) Mind Reacts to Sensations

What happens in the sixth stage of mind experience is an instinctive reaction to the changing biochemistry and hormones flooding through the body. Instinctive reactions can be to stop, attack, swear, run, embrace, cry, or smile. If someone were to threaten you with a gun, your mind perceives this as hostile and triggers the production of adrenaline; your breath stops and your heart pounds. Without even thinking, you run screaming for help or go on the attack. Alternatively, if your mind has triggered pleasant endorphins in reaction to a stimulus, you may react by wanting more. You might take another piece of cake, listen to a song one more time, go bungee jumping, or call a friend.

The moment before we react to biochemistry, whether it is creating a pleasant or an unpleasant sensation, is pivotal. In this split-second, we have the opportunity to change our behavior, and to change our habit-response. If we fail to exercise control, we simply react blindly, as we have always reacted in the past. If we do, we change nothing and our habitual behavior continues. It is in the moment before we react, however, that we can pause, examine, judge, observe, and think. This moment, gives us the opportunity to judge accurately and to act appropriately. By choosing our how we will act, speak, or even feel, we transform unhealthy behaviors and stop hurting others and ourselves with ignorant reactions. When we stop reacting blindly, and start living proactively, we become free.

7) Mind Stores a Conditioned Memory

The seventh stage of mind experience involves creating a memory. The mind remembers an experience and stores it away in its subconscious. The memory of an experience is more like a story than a series of images and information. Memories become complex analogies comprising a beginning, middle, and end. They have settings, characters, heroes, villains, plots, obstacles, and goals. A memory-story will also have meaning, relevance, and emotion. It comprises sensations, images, colors, sounds, smells, thoughts, judgments, relationships, movements, a sense of time and space, and beliefs. Each memory-story merges with a person's existing memories, changing and shaping the mind.

Remember the "snake" and all the feelings, sounds, shapes, and colors that were attached to the experience. You now know that a snake-like object could in fact, be a rope. You will recall the sensations of fear and relief. The next time you see a "snake" on the road you will think twice before reacting.

Throughout our lives, we continue to accumulate, build, and store countless memories that end up conditioning the way we think, feel, act, speak, understand, assume, and believe. As you can see, the more accurately we see things for what they really are, the less we will be conditioned by ignorance. The primary goal of practicing breath awareness is to train ourselves to stop, look, judge, choose our actions, and minimize ignorant conditioning.

Breath awareness trains us to hesitate, even for just a split second, before reacting to either a pleasant or an unpleasant sensation. If we can hesitate before reacting, and give ourselves time to objectively observe the thing, sensation, or event in question, we can make a proper judgment and act accordingly. Correct judgment allows us to choose how to respond and helps to ensure that the outcome will be positive and healthy.

We have now examined the stages that the mind goes through from perception to reaction. An object or thing comes into contact with one or more of our senses; mind perceives and becomes conscious of contact; the vibrations of the object or thing cause nerves to create a vibration, which is perceived as either pleasant, neutral, or unpleasant; mind recognizes the object or idea and passes judgment whether it is harmful or helpful; mind triggers an appropriate response by creating hormones or other natural chemicals; body, muscles, heart, nerves, and brain respond and react to these hormones; the memory of the experience is stored in the brain and merges into a pre-existing mental databank subsequently changing how we think.

As you can see, every experience goes through several stages before integrating and becoming part of the subconscious, or semi-conscious mind. How we process each stage of experience creates who we ultimately become. If we have misjudged situations and stored faulty information, we need to examine ourselves and try to find out what is true and what is false. Only then will we be able to acknowledge our false concepts, our misguided beliefs, our unwarranted fears, and make a radical change within ourselves.

Blind Reactions Lead to Developing Addictions

You may now be clear, at least intellectually, on how the brain triggers the production of brain and body chemicals in response to stimuli and how the mind then reacts to the pleasant or unpleasant sensations caused by these substances. You also understand that if you are unaware of what is happening inside your body, you develop cravings for pleasant hormones such as adrenaline, serotonin, or endorphins. You may now also understand how the mind craves pleasant sensations and can easily become addicted to them. Some things that we can become addicted to are hallucinogens, drugs, alcohol, nicotine, pornography, extreme sports, video games, caffeine, junk food, and gambling.

Let us look at another example of blind reaction. If a friend accuses you of lying, your mind registers the words as hostile, which triggers a flood of unpleasant sensations. In the past, before having trained your mind, you might have retaliated with harsh words. But this time, because you have developed mindmastery, you can stop, listen to the insults, and observe the painful sensations they create: blood rushes to your face, your eyes bulge, your eyes brim with tears, your lips quiver, your fists tighten. Now, with wisdom you acknowledge, *My friend is insulting me. No problem! The pain I feel is simply bodily sensations that cannot control me. I will stay calm and choose not to strike back at my ill-informed friend.*

When you are in control of blind reactions, you can exercise choice. Instead of lashing out with retaliatory words, sulking, or leaving the scene, you can calmly ask your friend to explain the problem and what he is feeling. If you develop the ability to stop reacting and rather start looking and listening, you will not only reduce conflict in your life, but you will have more freedom.

Becoming master of your mind means that you have control over blind reactions and unconscious cravings. You will not have control over the production of body and brain chemicals that produce pleasant sensations; however, you will have control over your reaction to sensations.

What Have You Learned About Your Mind?

- When you focus on breathing, your mind tends to wander.
- When your mind wanders, you can refocus on your breath.
- When your mind wanders, it is either thinking about the past or thinking about the future.
- When you hear a noise, you can keep your eyes closed.
- You know that breath is cool when you inhale.
- You know that breath is warm you exhale.
- You can choose to stay focused when you feel an ache.
- Some thoughts trigger feel-good sensations; others trigger unpleasant sensations.
- The more focused you are, the longer you can sit.
- The more focused you become, the less bored you feel.
- Habits have less control over you when you are focused.

You have learned many things about your mind and experienced how your happy, anxious, or sad thoughts can influence feelings. You are experiencing how different feelings are actually rooted in bodily sensations. Sadness, for example, may be rooted in a sensation of tightness in the chest or a strain in the head. Happiness may feel rooted in a sense of lightness in the heart area and an overall subtle vibration. Boredom may be rooted in a restricted feeling in the back or perhaps a dull throbbing in your head. Once you uncover the sensation connected to a feeling, use breath awareness to develop equanimity toward these thoughts, feelings, and sensations. After you have examined yourself in this way, resume feeling only the touch of breath.

Let us start again. We will do breath awareness for forty minutes in exactly the same way we have always practiced. However, in this session, as explained, we will observe the connection between our thoughts and the sensations that they generate. In this way, we can watch a sensation *before* it cause the habit-mind to react. See if you can feel a sensation before you react to it.

When your mind wanders, take note of what you are thinking before bringing yourself back to your breath. See if your thoughts are triggering feelings. This examination takes a second. Once you have noted your thought and its corresponding sensation, resume focusing on your breath. To perform this deep mind-examination, your mind must be extremely attentive.

Do not generate thoughts or conjure up images in your imagination. That is not your job. You will practice as always. The only difference is that when a thought does arise, acknowledge that a thought has arisen. Ask yourself, *What sensation am I feeling? Does this sensation correspond to this thought?* Once you are aware of the connection between your thought and your feeling or sensation, return to focusing on the breath.

Let us begin. Sit in a comfortable position. Keep your back straight. Close your eyes and fold your hands in your lap or rest them on your knees. We will be sitting for forty minutes. Start with a calm mind.

STUDENT PRACTICE SESSION (40 Minutes)

Fifteen-minute Silent Practice
Feel the incoming breath. Your natural, normal breath—as it is happening in the moment. When you feel your breath, you are feeling your present reality. Do not let one breath escape your attention. You are training your mind to be strong, alert, and attentive. You are not thinking about past things. You are not thinking about future events. You are experiencing the present moment.

Ten-minute Silent Practice
While moving to change position, continue observing your breath. If a thought pops into your mind, acknowledge the thought. Note if there is a corresponding sensation or feeling elsewhere on your body. Once you feel the sensation, go back to observing your breath.

Ten-minute Silent Practice
Stay alert and continue to focus on every single breath.

Five-minute Silent Practice - Session Concludes
You may open your eyes. No matter what thoughts arose or what sensations you experienced, let nothing disturb your peace. There is no need to feel disappointed or depressed. You have all successfully observed whatever feelings may have manifested in your mind and body without reacting to them. Congratulations, you worked very hard. It is time to relax and listen to another story.

PRINCE BLIND REACTION

There once lived a good-natured prince. One day, he received an invitation to attend a birthday celebration for the beautiful princess who lived in a neighboring kingdom. He instructed his humble servant, "Please, lay out my finest garments and ensure that my stallion is saddled and ready for an early departure. Tomorrow, I will be riding to the neighboring kingdom to attend a grand party."

Even before nightfall, the prince went to bed. He could not stop thinking about the princess and wanted to make sure he woke up early. He drank a cup of hot milk, donned his cozy pajamas, and because it was still light out, he slipped on his lightproof sleeping mask to help him get to sleep. Within minutes, he was dreaming about the princess.

The prince awoke before dawn. He sprang out of bed and groped around in the dark for his clothes. He pulled on his tights and silky vest and went downstairs. *Meeoooow!!* The prince tripped on something warm and fuzzy. It clawed at his leg as he tumbled down the hard marble steps. *"Ouch! Ouch! Ouch! Ouch!"* he cried.

The prince managed to find the castle door and once outside, he warily made his way to the stable. He bumped into his horse and groped for the reins. He felt nothing. His servant had forgotten to saddle up his horse. Instead of waiting around, he mounted the beast and commanded, "Onward, my trusty steed!" But his stallion wouldn't budge. Instead, it bucked wildly, until the prince toppled to the ground. "Ouch!" he whimpered, rubbing his broken ankle.

The sun still had not risen and the path was impossible to see. Worried that he would be late, the prince hobbled along. Thorn bushes and pointy branches scratched his face. "Oww!" he cried, flailing his arms and ripping prickly branches out of his way. The prince grew more determined; nothing would stop him from getting to the party. For several hours, he continued blindly limping ahead.

Finally, he arrived! Even though it was still pitch black, he felt the door and knocked loudly. While waiting, he imagined the beautiful princess and felt happy. The door opened. "Oh Prince, what have you done to yourself?" exclaimed a familiar voice. The prince was confused, "Am I not at the party? It's so dark. I can't see a thing." His trusty servant replied, "Your Highness, I'm terribly sorry, but you have arrived at your own castle. There is no party going on here. Might I ask, why are you wearing your sleeping mask in the middle of the day?"

The prince groped at his face and ripped off the mask. He squinted against the blinding daylight and peered around. What a shock! His hands were bleeding, his leg was scratched, his clothes were tattered, and his ankle was swollen. He looked outside and saw broken rose bushes strewn across the lawn. His cat, Fluffy, was licking her wound and the bull by the stable was still fuming mad. "What have I done?" the prince cried. The servant explained, "Prince, you forgot to remove your sleeping mask when you started on your journey."

The prince felt remorseful about the damage he had caused. He said sorry to his servant, hugged his cat, helped rake up the destroyed rose bushes, and consoled the angry bull. Most embarrassing of all, he sent a letter to the princess apologizing for his blind foolishness. The prince learned a lesson. From that day on, he made sure that nothing got in the way of seeing things clearly. Never again would he walk around with his sleeping mask covering his eyes and let his blind reaction hurt others and himself.

Student Journal

While making notes in your journal, consider these questions. Did you react blindly to something while sitting? Did you scratch an itch, or brush away a bug without first thinking? Did you feel restless and move around? When you felt a pain in your foot or back, could you wait a few moments and observe it before shifting your position? Did you feel any pleasant sensations? Could you observe the pleasant feelings and then go back to feeling your breath? Did you notice how your thoughts caused different feelings or emotions? If you stayed focused and observed a sensation, what happened? Did the sensation get more intense? Did it diminish?

Once you have noted your experiences, you may write your own story. It could be something about that happened to you in real life or something imagined. You can also illustrate your story or create a cartoon strip.

CHECK-IN

- Were you able to sit without moving despite pleasant or unpleasant sensations? Did you sometimes notice that you were craving, yearning, or wanting a particular sensation or feeling to happen?

- Did you want pain to subside? Could you acknowledge your craving or aversion and use the opportunity to develop equanimity toward the pleasant or unpleasant experience? Did you notice anger, resentment, depression, jealousy, doubt, or fear diminish while you were sitting?

- Were you able to observe how thoughts influence your state of mind and how your state of mind influences how you feel?

- Did you occasionally experience emotions such as sadness, disappointment, or worry? Could you acknowledge these emotions without reacting and then resume focusing on your breath?

- Did any emotions accumulate to an unbearable intensity? If so, could you stay calm? Did they eventually dissolve? Did this experience help you realize that all things, even emotions, change?

Continuation of Practice Tip: Even though breath awareness does not require you to change your diet, you might want to try a moderate cleansing or detoxifying diet. Cleansing your body of toxins will improve your focus and increase your well-being. It is more challenging to do breath awareness with a full stomach, therefore eat a lighter meal at night. As well, bowel elimination is important. Drink several glasses of water each day. A tablespoon of lemon or apple cider vinegar mixed with a glass of warm water is helpful.

STEP NINE

Freedom from Addiction

"Mindmastery has helped me so that I can master my thoughts and control my mind. We sat for forty minutes today and at the end, I was feeling restless. But I felt that I could control my mind and that I could use breath awareness in my daily life. I feel that I know how to do it. It is _not_ easy but it's _fun_!" —Jeremy, Age 10

YOUR PRACTICE SESSION - STEP NINE (60 Minutes)

The Importance of Sensation Awareness

Breath awareness is a mind-developing technique that uses sensation as its object of focus, where one's focus is restricted to a small area below the entrance of the nostrils. Observing sensation is the essence of the breath awareness technique. All sensation that occurs in this area, such as warmth, coolness, stinging, itchiness, vibrating, pulsating, and throbbing is included.

Many other "sensation awareness" techniques use sensation as their object of focus. Several of these, including breath awareness, will be described later in this chapter. Most of these methods share similar goals: to calm the mind; develop concentration; awaken self-awareness; purify mental defilements; overcome suffering; instill wisdom; generate compassion; and, ultimately enter into "enlightenment", the timeless, eternal state beyond experience.

Sensation is ideal to focus on for many reasons. The most important reason is that feeling sensation is a way to experience reality. Feeling sensation connects us with every vibrating square inch of ourselves.

Like breath, sensation is always with us. No matter where we go, no matter what we do, sensation will be there. The way to awaken awareness begins with consciously observing sensation from the moment you awake until the moment you fall asleep.

Generally, we are unaware of sensation. Think about the last time you drove your car, watched a movie, or ate dinner. Can you recall consciously feeling the particular sensations happening in your body during these activities? If you are like most of us, probably not. The danger is that if we do not awaken awareness sufficiently, we may eventually suffer a host of unwanted, uninvited problems.

When performing an activity without awareness, the unconscious, or subconscious mind freely shapes behavior. If a sensation is pleasant, the subconscious reacts with craving; if a sensation is unpleasant, it reacts with aversion. The subconscious is tirelessly feeling, communicating, responding, and reacting to sensations 24-7. The problem, therefore, is that if you are unconscious of sensation, you will also form habits unconsciously.

When unconsciously reacting to a sensation, the reaction influences and restructures the brain's neural circuitry because repetitive reactions influence how the brain is shaped. Eventually your unconscious actions become fixed neural networks, subsequently establishing your behavioral patterns. For these reasons, it is better to become conscious of sensation in order to prevent the subconscious from developing unhealthy behaviors, seemingly without your knowledge.

By consciously practicing an action, you are intentionally shaping your brain to achieve a desired skill, ability, habit, or behavior. The conscious repetition of an action, such as playing the guitar or operating a lathe, helps to acquire the ability to perform these actions more automatically. Unfortunately, the same principle applies to unhealthy behaviors, such as smoking or nail biting. If performed repetitively, the automatic behavioral patterns that are established are less desirable.

You might ask, "How do I prevent unconscious, unhealthy conditioning?" This question has perplexed humankind since first realizing how miserable life could be when one is controlled by unhealthy habits. At some point in history, around 5000 years ago, it was discovered that, mindfully observing the breath and sensations caused by the breath provided a way to at least minimize unconscious conditioning.

Observing sensation is probably the best measure for preventing unhealthy conditioning; and may be the best measure for cultivating behaviors that contribute to a more productive and healthy life.

Sensation is the Root of Experience
Sensation awareness is the key to cultivating behavior. As sensation is the root cause of experience, and experience is the root cause of behavior, it helps to analyze sensation in depth.

Without sensation, we would not feel emotion, fear, love, sexuality, inspiration, joy, intuition, or instinct. If we were void of sensation, we would not crave that which makes us feel good, or turn away from that which hurts. Craving and aversion are fundamental motivators for repeating a behavior, and therefore fundamental to shaping behavior.

Our reaction to pleasant and unpleasant sensations ultimately shapes who we become. Therefore, to undo or at least have some influence over how we behave, we may want to start consciously observing sensation.

Observing Sensation—A Way to Heal

Sensation awareness can heal unhealthy mental states. Anger, self-doubt, fear, hate, guilt, greed, depression, and anxiety are symptoms of unconsciously conditioned behavior. These states reveal that we have lost control and are allowing unhealthy habits to govern us.

Although sensation is always with us, and there is little reason not to be conscious of it, we have developed the habit of distracting ourselves from feeling it. When we go about our daily lives, we barely notice sensation. We may feel emotion, but emotion is a reaction and a symptom of underlying sensation. Just because we feel depressed, does not mean that we are conscious of the specific sensation causing our depression.

When sensations intensify, we have no choice but to be aware of them; however, by that time, they may be too painful to work with. Unfortunately, intense sensations such as pain or frustration may cause us to react, which may then lead to the formation of more unconscious behaviors. Reacting compromises the mind purification and transformative effect of any sensation awareness technique. Therefore, when practicing breath awareness, it is easier when the level of pain is tolerable.

Unraveling the Mystery of Impulsive Behavior

Most everything we think, feel, do, or say is governed by sensation, yet we are often clueless as to why we feel a specific emotion, or why we say or do certain things. Until we become conscious of the underlying sensations that cause our feelings and actions, we will not really grasp what is going on internally.

Observing sensation without reacting to it with craving or aversion develops equanimity. The very act of observing sensation non-reactively can effectively change both the sensation and one's habitual response to it. To illustrate non-reaction in practical terms, consider that the habit of smoking a cigarette when feeling nervous could be replaced by merely observing the sensation that is driving the desire to smoke. We might then observe that our hands are sweaty, our heart is throbbing, our chest is tightening, and our nerves are buzzing.

By remaining focused, we can continue observing the sensations and watch them change. We may note that nervousness intensifies, stays a while, and then gradually dissipates. Our heart may slow its pace, we may breathe more deeply, and our nervousness may lessen. Eventually, with no underlying sensations driving us to light a cigarette, we may decide not to smoke. In more severe addictions it might take a while before painful sensations dissolve, but eventually all sensations change; they arise, intensify, and then pass away—this is the nature of sensation.

Sensation helps us to "see" the unconscious or subconscious part of our mind that is responsible for shaping behavior. Sensation acts like a bridge connecting our conscious mind with the perplexing unconscious. Feeling sensation, therefore, is a way to experience, know, and transform who we are. Sensation leads us to the very root cause and source of our unhappiness.

Uprooting and Healing Unhealthy Memories

Sensation awareness provides a way to transform unhealthy memories and conditioning because when the mind is calm, unconscious memories tend to surface. When memories rise up, a dream or a past event may be remembered.

If memories surface when you are not in the middle of practicing breath awareness, they might cause you to start imagining and thinking. However, if they surface while doing breath awareness, you would merely continue focusing on your breath. This non-response would force the memory to manifest as a sensation, rather than as an image or thought, which is ideal. Once you *feel* something, you have a choice to either react or not to react to the feeling. By not reacting, you change your conditioned habit of reacting.

To illustrate this phenomenon, imagine that in order to suppress the emotional pain of an unhappy experience, you eat sugary comfort food. If you resist the craving, and instead practice breath awareness, you will observe that the pain may intensify and stay a while, but eventually it dissolves. Once the pain dissolves, so will your craving.

When focused exclusively on sensation, as you do while practicing breath awareness, a stream of memories is triggered and they surface. One after the next, memories pour from your subconscious. If you can refrain from intellectualizing or thinking about these memories, their accompanying sensations may intensify. In fact, any pain or unpleasantness may even manifest elsewhere in your body. Perhaps, for example, you also feel strain in your foot or pressure in your head.

When these sensations occur, stay focused on the sensation of breath. Although focusing might cause a particular sensation to intensify, eventually the pain will diminish and disappear. In this way, you can effectively uproot and rid your mind of unhealthy memories and, once gone, they no longer cause suffering.

Pain Manifests in our Weak Spots

When painful sensations manifest, they often do so in a weak joint or an old wound. When this manifestation happens, simply acknowledge the pain, and go back to the breath. It is of no real importance where pain manifests, nor does it matter what caused the pain. What is important is that pain has manifested, and that you are not reacting to it. By not reacting, you change your habit of reacting. However, should you lose focus and start thinking about the ailment or contemplating ways to relieve it, you will reinforce your conditioned behavior, which is counterproductive to your goal.

Observing sensation as a means to purify the mind and to eradicate unhealthy conditioning is not to be confused with psychotherapy. Breath awareness discourages imagining past events, talking about conceived problems, or performing any kind of self-analysis. Rather, the observation of sensation involves connecting to the root cause, the very biochemistry underlying a thought or memory. Breath awareness is an exercise of feeling, not intellectualizing.

There are many excellent and unique methods in use today to observe sensation. Mindfulness, or insight meditation, with its varied approaches, encompasses techniques that aim to develop an awareness of sensation. Although this book limits its instruction to the breath awareness technique, it is helpful to understand other methods of sensation awareness, as you may want to explore them in the future. The methods are all very similar to breath awareness and they may even help expand your capacity to observe sensation. The greater your capacity, the more you will experience your inner self.

Despite the wonderful benefits that come from sensation awareness techniques when practiced by adults, most of the intense and serious exercises are not suitable for children. Teaching a variety of techniques to children would compromise the effect of doing breath awareness well. In fact, if instructed to fix their attention on bodily sensations other than those caused by the breath, children might experience undue psychological or emotional upheaval. Children can achieve safe and proven results by practicing breath awareness exclusively.

The following descriptions simply aim to provide a brief overview of some of the methods of observing sensation. If interested in practicing one or more of these methods, it is highly recommended that you learn the techniques properly, under the guidance of a qualified teacher. Again, I emphasize the importance of not mixing techniques, especially when teaching children.

Eight Methods for Observing Sensation

1) Observing Sensations of Breath (Breath Awareness)

Observing sensations of breath involves fixing the attention in and around the nose and feeling sensation caused by breath touching the skin. In this particular technique, focus is limited to a small area directly around the nostrils. When practiced correctly, breath awareness can lead to all stages of mind development and experience. The technique can calm the mind, reduce stress, strengthen concentration, awaken awareness, generate compassion, and ultimately lead one to attaining the timeless, eternal state beyond sensation experience. Breath awareness, therefore, is a complete technique in and of itself. As well, it is a safe and effective exercise for children.

2) Observation of Randomly Occurring Sensations

Observation of randomly occurring sensations involves a passive mindfulness of the body and mind. When a sensation or thought presents itself, the practitioner directs the attention toward it and spends a few minutes observing its changing characteristics. After examining the sensation or thought, another sensation may arise. The attention turns toward this new event and objectively observes it. This technique also uses mind states and emotions such as anger, sadness, stress, fatigue, boredom, or joy to focus on. When a painful or pleasurable emotion floods through the body, the practitioner acknowledges the feeling without developing craving or aversion toward it. Being mindful of randomly occurring thoughts, sensations and emotions helps to calm and focus the mind, release tension, develop equanimity and acceptance of one's reality, and generate loving kindness toward whatever pleasant or unpleasant sensations arise.

3) Part-by-part Observation of Surface Sensations

Part-by-part observation of surface sensations involves a methodical examination of the body's surface sensations—one square inch at a time. The practitioner fixes attention on this small area until a sensation is felt.

Once a sensation manifests, the attention moves on to examine the adjacent square inch. If none is felt, the practitioner focuses for a minute or two longer before continuing. Each time the attention returns to this insensitive area, it again tries to detect sensation. By repeatedly returning to examine the numb area, eventually a sensation will start to vibrate. In this technique, all sensations, whether pleasant, neutral, or unpleasant, share equal importance and include tingling, throbbing, heat, coolness, stinging, sweat, prickling, strain, and pressure.

To perform a full-body part-by-part scan, the practitioner starts examining the top of the head. Then, in a systematic manner, travels down to the forehead, eyebrows, eyes, nose, cheeks, lips, ears, neck, shoulders, arms, elbows, hands, fingers, torso, back, legs, knees, and toes. Once a downward part-by-part scan is completed, the practitioner performs the meticulous examination in reverse. Any downward or upward route is acceptable, provided no areas are missed.

Systematic observation ensures that the attention passes over all areas, even those that are numb, blind, or insensitive. The goal is to connect consciousness with every part of the body, leaving no part unobserved. A full part-by-part examination from head to toe might take twenty to forty minutes. As the attention becomes alert, and all numb spots have been activated, a complete scan will take less time.

Part-by-part observation can calm the mind, sharpen attention, and awaken awareness. When the body is free of numb areas, and gross sensations of pain and pressure have dissolved, the practitioner may feel a flow of subtle energy. This intensive, penetrating, observation of sensations is not suitable for children, as it can trigger a flow of suppressed and traumatic memories or cause unpleasant physical reactions.

4) Part-by-part Observation of Internal Sensations

Part-by-part observation of internal sensations is similar to the method just described, yet this time the practitioner examines sensations occurring internally. Sensations are felt in the brain, eyeballs, inner ear, mouth, veins, bones, muscles, and organs such as the stomach and heart.

An internal part-by-part examination starts in the brain. The attention then weaves from one side of the head, through the brain, to the other. Attention can also travel from the back of the head toward the front. Alternatively, the attention can travel in a circular fashion that spirals downward through the entire body. Although there is no particular path that the attention must follow, traveling the same route prevents inadvertently skipping over a blind area. To clarify, the internal scan is not an imaginary journey through one's body; there are no mental images of the heart or brain. The journey progresses one sensation to the next sensation.

A serious, penetrating part-by-part internal examination can also trigger unconscious states that might overwhelm a person who is practicing on their own. It is advisable, therefore, that this scanning technique be practiced under the guidance of an experienced teacher. As well, it is not a suitable technique for young people.

5) Observing Surface Sensation by Sweeping

Observing surface sensation by sweeping is another way to feel sensation. This method requires the practitioner to "sweep" the attention over a section of the body, for example, the neck, chest, and stomach. Or, it can be used to sweep the entire body, with a single pass. To perform a sweep, the attention moves over the selected area feeling all sensations in its path.

To perform a full body sweep (sometimes called a "body scan"), attention starts by focusing at the top of the head. Once sensation is felt, the attention is directed to move down over the whole body similar to taking a shower. As attention moves downward, it feels sensations along the way.

To be clear, sweeping is not an exercise of the imagination; one does not visualize standing under a shower and "seeing" water pouring over the body. Rather, the attention *feels* the experience. As attention moves over the skin's surface, sensations are actually felt. Sweeping can also be performed when one is lying down and works best when the mind is calm and the body is free of gross sensation. The aim of this technique is to experience the whole body as one vibrating mass of subtle energy.

6) Observing Internal Sensation by Sweeping

Observing internal sensation by sweeping is a similar method to the one described above. Only this time, the attention moves with one flowing motion through either a section inside body, for example, through the lungs, heart, and stomach, or it moves through the body from the head to the toes. The sweep can also be a gentle movement, like ink dropping into water; the awareness flows down naturally, spreading and dispersing into every part of the body. Sweeping is best performed when the mind is calm and there are no gross sensations present.

7) Checking for Numb Areas

Checking for numb areas is a technique used to ensure that the body has no areas void of sensation. To perform a random check, the practitioner focuses attention on a selected point, such as in the finger, earlobe, or toe. After feeling a sensation, the attention moves on to check another spot. If no sensation is felt, the practitioner continues to fix the attention there. If, after a minute or two, there is still no sensation, the practitioner proceeds checking other points, now and again, returning to check this numb area.

8) Observing Sensation while Performing Activities

Observing sensation while performing activities offers a way to develop mindfulness throughout the day. One method involves being mindful of sensations that happen when doing a normal, natural movement or activity, such as walking, feeling rain or wind against the face, listening to music, waiting for a bus, or swimming. The practitioner simply observes whatever sensation manifests. This could be feeling sensation in one body part or the whole body.

The other way involves slowing down the activity and performing an intensive examination of each sensation that occurs. For example, in a practice known as *walking meditation*, a practitioner would slow walking to a snail's pace. Each step is performed with mindfulness. The meditation often starts with standing. The practitioner is mindful of all the sensations caused by standing. Then, he or she would raise the foot and feel sensations caused by this movement. With each step, the practitioner is mindful of sensations caused by the weight of the foot; the strain of the working muscle, the stretching leg; and the impact of stepping down. The exercise may involve only twenty or thirty steps in a one-hour session.

Similarly, this method of observing sensation can be applied to eating, sitting, or lying down. In fact, any normal, ordinary activity can become the object of a sensation awareness meditation.

When you investigate different meditation or mind-development methods, you will find that many incorporate breath awareness together with one or more of the above techniques. The reason for mentioning different techniques at this stage of your practice is to emphasize the importance of sensation. As well, it may help to know that what you have been learning encompasses the fundamental principles of these other more "advanced" practices.

Several of the more intense sensation awareness techniques are described as "deep operations of the mind". When practiced seriously, they can trigger a release of emotional or psychological trauma, or unpleasant sensations. The practitioner may experience heat, shaking, trembling, numbness, burning, or intense emotions of fear or sadness. Because of the intensity of such techniques, you might feel more confident learning and practicing them under the guidance of a properly trained teacher in a suitable environment. If you become interested in learning one of these techniques, you will find many opportunities to do so. There are numerous mindfulness and vipassana meditation retreats offered worldwide.

Your Practice Session – Step Nine
Start this one-hour session with a calm and attentive mind. Sit erect, close your eyes, and focus your attention entirely on your incoming and outgoing breath. Remind yourself that you are not wasting your time; rather, you are expanding a dimension of your life, investigating your inner reality, and gaining valuable experience.

In this sitting, become aware of all sensation caused by the breath. Keep your attention firmly fixed on whatever sensation arises. Stay with each sensation and observe what happens. Start with feeling sensation inside your nose. After a few minutes, move your attention to the entrance of your nostrils. Feel the cool and warm breath pass over this area. Finally, narrow your focus to a tiny spot just below the entrance of your nostrils. Keep your entire attention firmly fixed on this one spot without letting yourself become distracted. Try not to miss a single breath. Acknowledge any sensations that arise on this spot.

Remember, sensations provide the opportunity to develop equanimity. Sensations connect you with your present-moment reality and provide a bridge to your unconscious mind. Sensations are the root cause of every experience, and by consciously observing them you are consciously experiencing your reality, as it is happening in the present moment. Your experience of molecular vibrations and energy will help you realize your true, changing nature. You will realize that nothing stays the same, nothing is fixed, nothing is permanent, and that all life, including yours, is perpetually changing. This is reality.

Wherever you fix your attention, whether inside your nose, at the entrance of your nostrils, or under your skin, remain aware of the sensation's changing characteristics. Be mindful of your breath's rhythm, its temperature, its shallowness, or deepness. Be mindful of the exact moment your mind perceives the in-breath touching your skin. Be mindful of the breath's touch as it passes over your skin. Then be mindful of the absence of breath on the skin. Repeat the same examination of your out-breath.

While feeling breath, be aware of your entire physical structure. Experience the subatomic flow of energy as it vibrates throughout your body. Be mindful of your entire mental construct, its contents, imagination and ideas. Be a witness to how your transient thoughts arise, stay a while, and eventually dissipate.

Remember that the key to success in effecting real transformation is to remain objective and non-reactive toward any sensation, whether painful, neutral, or pleasant. Be like a scientist who objectively investigates the natural laws governing mind and matter. As such, you will unravel the mysteries of who you are.

Observing sensation, whether caused by your breath, or manifesting on other parts of your body, is a way to experience your physical and mental reality as it is happening in the present moment. Sometimes your reality will feel uncomfortable; other times it will feel pleasant and energized. Even when experiencing blissful vibrations, your job remains the same—to keep scanning, investigating, penetrating, and becoming more conscious of your reality.

When pleasant sensations cause you to crave, or when you feel pain and start wanting the pain to go away, remember that craving and aversion are counterproductive to developing equanimity and realizing your Truth. When your session is over, you may wish to reflect on the questions in Your Check-in.

TEACHER TIPS

Our unconscious craving or aversion to a particular sensation is the root cause of all addictions. To become free, one must consciously and continuously examine the sensation with an equanimous mind. —Attributed to Buddha

Observing Mind States with Equanimity

Congratulations on your efforts! The hard work of learning the breath awareness technique and how to teach children is done. You have inspired your students to work correctly and encouraged them to work seriously. You may have experienced many meaningful moments since you first started the program and your efforts have certainly given children a precious life-changing experience.

In this session, students will be sitting for forty-five minutes. They will learn to recognize how an addiction or habit begins, how it continues, and how to break free from its control. Addictions, as we all know, can be the most debilitating condition that a person, young or old, develops. Many of us, in fact, have minor addictions. Perhaps we are compulsive chocolate or caffeine consumers and some of us might even suffer a serious drug, gambling, or pornography addiction. Serious addictions can destroy one's health, relationships, and happiness.

Unfortunately, humans are habit-forming creatures. Although some habits help us survive, others are self-defeating. Healthy habits, like exercising, drinking water, or brushing one's teeth generally have life-sustaining, positive outcomes. However, when habits become harmful or unhealthy they become addictions. When we are addicted we become slaves to our habit-mind. We lack the will power to make choices or to implement them. Our minds become weak and dull and it becomes even more difficult to know what is healthy. The aim of breath awareness is to strengthen the mind so it is less susceptible to forming addictions.

Dealing with Emotions

It is important to understand what your students experience while they practice breath awareness. Although one can never know what students are actually thinking and feeling, it is safe to make assumptions based on your observations. When a student has attained a degree of focus and is sitting for longer periods, for example, he or she may experience an upsurge of suppressed memories that manifest as a thoughts, emotions, or sensations.

For a beginner student this experience may be overwhelming. When traumatic "memory-seeds" manifest as sensation, the student will become aware of increased discomfort either in one part or in his or her whole body. While teaching, you might notice a child weeping, trembling, or making contorted facial expressions. These behaviors are often signs that suppressed emotions are surfacing. Children should be assured that when suppressed memories manifest as physical sensations or painful emotions, it indicates that the technique is working.

Although these manifestations are signs of progress, remind children not to focus on bodily sensations, as this focus will intensify the pain. Focusing on bodily sensations is an advanced technique for adults, as explained in Step Nine. Practicing intense sensation awareness is not appropriate for children so we try to keep the child's attention fixed only on the touch of breath.

Even if we continually remind students to stay focused on the small area of skin at the entrance of their nostrils, many will still feel sensation elsewhere. They may have a headache, sore stomach, numb leg, or feel light-headed and dizzy. Whenever you see a student paying attention to bodily sensations, remind him or her to go back to focusing on the breath.

Some children write in their journals about feeling bodily sensations. When you read what they have written, you will have an idea of what is going on and can remind them to stay fixed on the breath. By encouraging focused attention, you will ensure that students work on the surface of their minds, preventing traumatic or emotional issues from arising.

It is not that we want children to avoid dealing with psychological problems. Rather, a classroom environment is just not appropriate, particularly when a student has to go somewhere right after their breath awareness session—maybe to a hockey game or a daycare. If a sensitive child has triggered unresolved issues, abrupt confrontation with noisy, external distractions could do more harm than good.

Children are complex beings with more buried in them than meets the eye. If something comes up and you feel unqualified to deal with it, talk to the child's parent or refer the child to a school guidance counselor.

Addiction is Rooted in Sensation and Memory

Humans seem governed less by reason and rational thinking, and more by emotions and feelings. It is hard to override feelings, as they cause a person to feel a certain way—usually good or bad. Emotions are rooted in sensations; sensations caused by our body's reactions to its biochemistry. Anger can result when the body produces an abundance of adrenaline and testosterone, but lacks sufficient serotonin, the happy hormone. Depression may be caused by our reaction to unpleasant sensations caused by the body's lack of norepinephrine, dopamine, and serotonin.

It would help to understand how brain chemistry is produced, how it triggers sensation, and ultimately, how sensation creates emotion. Without awareness of this physiological chain of events, our behavior and feelings will be controlled by sensation.

From the moment of conception until the moment of death our six sense doors—eyes, ears, mouth, nose, skin, and mind—come into contact with infinite visual, audible, and sensory stimuli and vibrations including light, sound, color, taste, smell, and feeling. Before we feel a sensation, our minds must detect or perceive one or more of these vibrations. Sometimes these vibrations feel good; other times they feel painful.

After the mind experiences a particularly pleasant vibration, for example, the memory of this enjoyable feeling causes the mind to want to repeat the experience. The memory causes the mind to start craving this particular sensation and you find yourself saying, *I want more.* Similarly, if the sensation is uncomfortable or painful, the mind develops aversion toward it, and you find yourself saying, *I do not want more.*

Repeating experiences and developing habits can be useful. In nature, animals, like humans, create complex behavior and habit patterns based on their reactions to pleasure or pain. These habits become ingrained and instinctual, and often promote survival. Ironically, our human instinctual ability to develop life-sustaining habits can also lead to developing harmful, life-threatening habits.

The problem with humans is our incredible ability to remember, imagine, and project into the future. Our imaginations can conjure up past pleasures and then imagine receiving those pleasures again in the future. This imaginary projection of receiving something pleasant creates craving. A person who is depressed, for example, may remember how much better it felt to eat chips or to smoke a cigarette, and may then start craving these things. As well, if we have had the experience of pain, our memory will cause us to do whatever it takes to avoid repeating the painful experience in the future.

We spend considerable time suppressing pain or evoking pleasure. If we feel depressed and perhaps start eating chips or light up a cigarette, we temporarily suppress pain. These substances stimulate the production of pleasure hormones and neurotransmitters like serotonin and dopamine, which help dull the intensity of the pain. Because these aids cause us to feel better, our memory wants to repeat the experience. To sustain a pain-free state, we either keep eating until the bag of chips is empty or smoking until the whole pack of cigarettes is gone.

Craving and aversion happen in virtually every area of our lives. We always want more of something. We want more things, friends, money, fame, recognition, compliments, companionship, security, sex, health, or power. We crave adrenaline-induced excitement, dangerous sports, mind-numbing alcohol, or heart-throbbing violence. We yearn for love, comfort, respect, peace, acceptance, or spiritual experiences.

Of course many things like love, appreciation, peace, respect, and acceptance are fundamental to our emotional, mental, and spiritual well-being. We all need a safe place to live, food to keep us alive, and a loving relationship we can depend on. However, the problem occurs when we start craving and wanting. Craving creates insatiable dissatisfaction and unending suffering. To be happy, we must recognize our needs, fulfill them the best we can, enjoy pleasures and comforts, but be cautious not to develop craving.

Craving Underlies Addiction

How does craving lead to addiction? Remembering something pleasurable triggers the mind to start craving. We are then compelled to indulge in whatever caused the pleasant or stimulating sensation in the past. We repeat the same action, and again experience the sought after pleasant sensation. The urge often happens at the unconscious level of the mind, making it difficult to control or stop.

The more we repeat the action, the more obsessed we become and as we continue to overindulge in the substance or activity, we tax our health. Our habit-mind takes control and we are powerless to stop. When we cannot stop indulging in a harmful substance or activity, we have become addicted.

By practicing breath awareness, we can isolate and become conscious of the very sensation that is causing our craving. Then, through objective examination of the sensation, we can become aware of the source of our craving. Becoming aware is the first step to gaining control and changing harmful habits. Our goal is not to suppress or escape pleasant or unpleasant sensation, nor is it to suppress or deny the experience of sensation. Our task lies in becoming conscious of the root cause of craving, namely sensation.

STUDENT INSTRUCTIONS - STEP NINE

Freedom from Addiction

Welcome to your ninth session of Mindmastery. You have been practicing seriously. Your mind is alert; your attention is sharp. Your examination of your mind and body has given you valuable self-knowledge and many other insights. You have learned how to observe your breath. You have also experienced sensations in other parts of your body, acknowledged them, and refocused on your breath.

You have experienced that some days you feel calm or happy; other days you feel sad or restless. You have learned that boredom, indifference, and apathy are also feelings, though disagreeable. You have learned how to examine your feelings and how to uncover their underlying sensations. You have experienced that sensation can be pleasant, neutral, or unpleasant. You have gained self-discipline and have remained calm despite unpleasant sensation. All these discoveries and skills indicate that you are developing more awareness, working properly, and cultivating mindmastery.

Most of you have experienced how your thoughts affect your feelings and how your feelings affect your thoughts. This is an important observation. Exciting thoughts make you feel good. Sad thoughts make you feel unhappy. Thoughts and feelings are two sides of the same coin; heads is feeling and sensation, tails is thought and imagination. One minute you are feeling sensation; the next minute, you are thinking about something in your mind.

Your attention jumps constantly from thinking to feeling and back again. Your mind has been jumping around from the moment you were born and will continue jumping around until the moment you die. By learning how to master your mind you are learning how to control the jumping around. This mental discipline will give you the power to focus, which will help you achieve your goals. You are becoming aware of how easy it is to get addicted to a thought. Because you enjoy the sensation that a particular thought causes, you keep thinking the thought over and over again. You know that it is not the thought you are addicted to, but the sensation attached to it. While doing breath aware-ness, you may suddenly recognize the particular sensation you are ad-dicted to. Once you see the underlying cause of your addiction, you will understand that you are not addicted to the thought; rather, you are addicted to the sensation that the thought creates.

For instance, the emotion of revenge can be addictive; for example, you might feel revenge toward a person and become obsessed with getting back at that person. You spend your days and nights thinking about what the person did to you and keep thinking of ways to punish him or her. Your thoughts of revenge generate more anger, which in turn fuels your revenge. In this way, you keep your revenge burning. It is through this process that you become addicted to your rage and may even begin enjoying the fiery, adrenaline-pumped feeling. Unless you become con-scious of what is happening, though, you may lose control and end up hurting someone. If you hurt anyone, your actions will ultimately end up harming you; your mind will become agitated and you will have no peace.

Practicing breath awareness provides the mental stillness needed to observe the sensations of rage and anger. Your practice allows you to sit calmly, watch, wait, and wisely assess a situation. With composure, you can then choose what action you will take. In other words, you will gain control. This control allows you to choose how to react. If you can con-trol your unconscious and ignorant reactions to sensation, you will avoid addiction. As you gain mastery over your impulsive, addictive habit-mind, you will find it easier to control yourself. Do not worry about *trying* to control yourself. Change happens when you practice.

How do Addictions Start?
As long as your habits give you pleasure or suppress pain, you will probably continue doing whatever it is that makes you feel good. If your habits are unhealthy and gradually dull or damage your mind or body, eventually you will suffer. Unfortunately, some habits are hard to break, even when you realize they are harmful.

Let's look at a common situation, one that many have experienced, to investigate how habits end up controlling behavior. Your doctor tells you that you cannot eat your favorite food, French fries, because you are overweight, have high blood pressure, and are at risk for a heart attack. You promise the doctor that you will not to eat any more fries. The next day you tell yourself, *I promise, from this day forward, not to eat any fries.*

The first day passes and you avoid eating fries! The second day is more difficult, but you refrain, and feel great about yourself. However, on the third day someone makes an insensitive remark about your weight or looks. The words hurt and you are overcome with feelings of depression, loneliness, and self-doubt. You feel so miserable that all you want is for the pain to go away. Without thinking, you order fries. *Yummy! They taste so good!* While eating them you feel less miserable; eating numbs the pain. When this happens, your unconscious habit-mind breathes a sigh of relief, *Now I feel better.* To keep the pain away and maybe even to punish yourself for your lack of willpower, you keep eating. Soon, you become physically ill. Your habit-mind cannot tolerate emotional or physical pain so it suppresses the hurt by eating more, despite the doctor's orders.

Now you suffer regret, remorse, and guilt. You start thinking that you are weak-willed and will always be overweight. You even begin hating yourself. These self-defeating thoughts cause your mind to produce biochemistry that makes you feel worse. You try to combat the feeling with more fatty food but the downward spiral continues and your addiction to fries perpetuates. How will you break this cycle of emotional addiction?

When we make a decision to do something, we are using our "thinking" mind. For example, you tell yourself, *I will study hard for the exam.* However, when you sit down to study, restlessness overwhelms you. This is your unconscious habit-mind at work. Unless you spend time mastering your voluntary attention and transforming your ingrained conditioning, your conscious mind will never be stronger than your habit-mind.

The best way to gain mindmastery and be stronger than your habit-mind is to practice breath awareness and to train your voluntary attention. You will be glad to know that for the past eight Mindmastery sessions, that is exactly what you have been doing—diligently training your voluntary attention. Every minute that you sat calmly observing breath, you were strengthening your attention. Every time you refrained from reacting to unpleasant sensations, restlessness, or agitation, you were gaining control over your habit-mind. Some of you may have noticed changes in your behaviors and habits over the past few days; maybe you fidget less; maybe you focus better. Maybe you have stopped biting your nails, reaching for your iPod, or eating junk food. These changes indicate that you are breaking your habits and gaining control over your choices and actions.

We only have one more breath awareness session to practice seriously before Mindmastery is over. Use your time wisely; use every minute to develop your focus and attention. Let us begin. Sit comfortably with your back and neck straight. Direct your attention to the touch of breath as it enters and leaves your nose. We will be sitting for forty-five minutes.

STUDENT PRACTICE SESSION (45 Minutes)

Ten-minute Silent Practice
Start with a calm and peaceful mind. Feel your cool natural breath as it comes in. Feel your warm natural breath as it goes out. Observe every single breath as it is. There is no need to control the breath. Observe your reality as it happens. Let not one breath escape your attention. This is how you train your mind to become strong, alert, and attentive.

Ten-minute Silent Practice
Limit your area of focus to a small point just below your nose. The smaller the area, the more focused you will become. Breathe in. Breathe out. If you feel agitated, know that you are agitated, and refocus on your breath.

Five-minute Silent Practice
If you feel restless, stay focused on your breath. If you feel pain, acknowledge, *Oh, I feel pain.* Then focus on your breath. If there is a distraction or if your mind wanders, acknowledge, *Oh, my mind has wandered.* Resume focusing on your breath. Restlessness has no power over you. You may experience a pleasant sensation. You may experience an unpleasant sensation. You may experience a neutral sensation. Do not let any sensation distract you from feeling your breath.

If you become aware that you are craving a particular sensation, realize that you have become distracted. You might hear your mind saying, *I am uncomfortable; I want to get up. I do not like the pain in my foot. I want to get rid of my headache. I want something to eat. I feel bored. I want this feeling to go away.*

This is your habit-mind talking. Acknowledge that your mind is craving, and resume focusing on your breath. Breath awareness is about observing what is happening in the present moment, not about wanting this thing or that thing to happen. Focus on your breathing. Feel the breath as it passes over the small area below your nostrils and above your upper lip. Breathe in. Breathe out with awareness. Continue training your attention to stay on one small spot.

Ten-minute Silent Practice

Breathe in. Breathe out. If you are tired, take a few hard breaths and then resume with natural, normal breathing. Straighten your back. Stay alert. Resume normal breathing. If your mind has wandered, acknowledge it and then bring it gently back to the breath.

Keep your eyes closed; opening your eyes will break your focus. Be alert and attentive. Be perfectly still, perfectly balanced. Let nothing disturb your equanimity.

Ten-minute Silent Practice - Session Concludes

Good work! You may open your eyes. If you wish to change your position, you may do so. If you wish to continue listening to the story with closed eyes, you may choose to do so.

You are developing control over your habit-mind. You are no longer craving sensation, whether pleasant or unpleasant, exciting or boring. Sensation cannot control you. Your conscious mind is strong and your semi-conscious habit-mind has no power. You are becoming the master of your mind. It is again time for a story.

I Want the Moon!

There once lived a caring couple who were about to have a baby. It was a joyous day when their son was born and they named him Morpli. Morpli was a quiet and peaceful baby and his parents proudly told their friends, "Morpli is the best baby ever; he never ever cries." Their friends nodded, "Is that so?"

A few days later, they heard a faint *"whaa"* coming from the crib. The mother said, "Is that Morpli?" Nodding, the father replied, "Maybe he's hungry." She gave him some milk and he stopped crying. The parents sighed relief, but after a few minutes they heard a louder *"whaa, whaa."* "What could he want now?" asked Mom. Dad suggested, "Maybe he's cold?" They wrapped Morpli in a blanket and he calmed down; however, twenty minutes later they heard him cry, *"Whaa, whaa."*

The parents guessed that Morpli needed to be changed. After Morpli was clean and dry, he smiled. But soon his smile turned to tears. Morpli had to burp. Finally, after Morpli was fed, changed, burped, and tucked into bed, he closed his eyes and was quiet. His parents sat down to rest, but moments later they heard *"whaa, whaa."* What did Morpli want now? Mom lovingly lifted him out of the crib and rocked him in her arms. Morpli felt warm, safe, loved, and happy and soon fell fast asleep.

The next morning mom and dad awoke to a familiar *"whaa, whaa."* They sprang to work, knowing exactly what to do. They fed, changed, burped, and gently rocked little Morpli until he fell asleep. For the following months this became their daily routine and Morpli was happy. One day, the parents heard Morpli cry louder than ever. He was reaching for his teddy bear; but when Mom handed him Teddy, he continued crying. Oh, he probably wants Monkey. When Morpli got his monkey stuffy, he calmed down. Mom and Dad became experts in knowing exactly what their son wanted.

Eighteen months later, Morpli could walk and talk. One day, dad heard a loud, "Owww!" Morpli had fallen down. His father hugged him, put a bandage on his knee, and offered him ice cream. After his son had eaten a whole bowl full, he looked up at his dad and cried, *"More plea, Dada, more plea."* Dad gave him more and Morpli was happy. After that day, whenever Morpli hurt himself he wanted ice cream.

The older Morpli got the more things he wanted. On his fifth birthday, he received a tricycle. While happily riding down the sidewalk, his buddy who lived next door, rode up on a shiny two-wheeler with motorcycle handlebars. Morpli stared enviously at his buddy's bike and looked with dismay at his childish tricycle. That evening, Morpli begged his parents for a bike with motorcycle handlebars.

On his next birthday, Morpli received a cool bike with special handle-bars. After that, there was no end to things that Morpli wanted.

For his ninth birthday he begged, "I want a Combat 3 DVD." When he was ten he whined, "I want an iPod." At twelve he pleaded, "May I have a laptop with 3-D apps." At fifteen he argued, "I want a scooter." At sixteen he insisted, "How about a car, Dad?" Dad thought that fixing up a car would be a learning opportunity for his teenage son and bought a broken-down Volvo. With Dad's help, Morpli fixed up the old car and proudly drove it school. Something zoomed past him at lightning speed. It was his buddy in a sports car with the beautiful Angelina sitting next to him. Morpli thought, "Volvos are for old folks, I want a sports car." He got a job and leased a high-powered, metallic blue racing car.

Morpli happily drove around town, but despite having the ultimate ve-hicle, he felt that something was missing. "If only I had a girlfriend," he sighed. Not too long after, he fell in love with a nice girl who really liked him. They drove around in his car and life rocked. All Morpli wanted was a higher paying job so he attended university and earned a degree. After graduation, he had everything a young man could want—a degree, a girl-friend, a car, and parents who were proud of him.

Morpli wanted his wonderful life to continue and contemplated, "If I married my sweetheart, I would be happy for the rest of my life." A few years later, he married, bought a house, and worked at a high-salary job. Despite having everything he wanted, he felt dissatisfied. He thought that children would make him happy. The couple were blessed with a daughter, and later, two sons. Morpli then wanted a bigger house, a SUV, and a dog. Everyone thought that Morpli's life was perfect. Nevertheless, Morpli still felt unhappy.

Morpli worked long hours and felt worn out. He wanted to feel better so he bought a holiday house, installed two wide-screen TVs, and hired a nanny. Despite these luxuries, he felt stressed and started to smoke. His doctor advised, "Morpli, you must stop smoking, you are getting addicted. Take a vacation." Morpli went to Mexico, bought a motorboat, a Sea-doo, and a seaplane. He took pills to calm down and sleep better. But, no matter what he tried, no matter how many vacations he went on, nothing made him happy.

One day Morpli read an advertisement: Every Man Needs a Private Rocket Ship. He thought, "Oh, a rocket ship, now that's what I *really* want. Why didn't I think of this in the first place?" Morpli mortgaged all he owned and put a down payment on a rocket ship. Then he thought, "What good is a rocket ship unless I can go somewhere in it?" He looked up into the night sky and gazed longingly at the beautiful moon. "I want to go to the moon. No, actually, *I want the moon!*" "Sorry Morpli, you cannot have the moon," said a representative from NASA, the organization that controls the US space program. Morpli sighed, "I would rather die than not have the moon." Morpli obsessed over the moon. His psychiatrist could not make him stop wanting it.

Morpli was now ninety years old and very ill. He lay in the hospital bed, surrounded by his family. He kept moaning, "I want the moon. I want the moon." His family listened, sadly shaking their heads. Unable to get what he wanted, Morpli closed his eyes. He felt his cool breath come in through his nose. He felt his warm breath go out of his nose. For hours, he kept breathing in and breathing out. He felt a sense of oneness with everything; as if he was part of the whole universe. His obsessive wanting started to fade. As it disappeared, he no longer wanted the moon. With the wanting gone, he felt different.

Morpli opened his eyes and saw his family watching over him. As he looked at his beautiful wife and children, he realized that he had spent his whole life wanting and wanting. Nothing could have satisfied this insatiable craving. His daughter noticed her father's expression change and asked, "Dad, are you OK? Do you want something?" Morpli smiled, "No, nothing. I want nothing at all." Morpli reached for his daughter's hand. For the first time in his life his heart felt full of love and happiness. He closed his eyes and peacefully passed away.

When we are young and dependent, we need our parents' love, care, attention, and protection. This is normal, natural, and necessary. When we mature, we turn our attention away from our own survival and find joy in taking care of others, our partner, children, and community. However, we may have unknowingly become addicted to the sensation of wanting. When this happens, nothing can truly satisfy us. Even when we get everything we want, we still want more. When Morpli stopped wanting, he got everything and was finally happy.

Student Journal

Describe your experience, noting your different feelings and thoughts that you had while doing breath awareness. You can also write or draw a story about wanting or craving something. It can be a real story imagined; it can be serious or humorous. Write whatever you think will best express what you have learned so far. You might like to include in your story how the main character overcomes his or her wanting or addiction. Later, we can share our stories with each other. Have fun!

CHECK-IN

- After feeling calm and pleasant, did waves of deeper agitation surface?

- Did any unpleasant sensations interrupt your breath awareness practice? Could you stay focused on breathing?

- While practicing breath awareness, did you feel sensations in other parts of your body? Could you return to your breath?

- Could you remain calm and observe arising sensations without reacting and then return to your breath?

- Were you aware of vibrations throughout your entire body? Where they pleasant or unpleasant?

- Did you experience how everything is moving, vibrating, and changing inside your body?

Continuation of Practice Tip: You may be interested in joining a ten-day sensation awareness retreat. You will find this technique called by different names such as Mindfulness Meditation, Insight or vipassana meditation. Do your research, ask others about what they have experienced, and discover which technique seems most suitable for you. Most meditation courses are free of charge and are supported by donations. If you have little funds, many will let you join anyway. Remember that breath awareness is also a serious technique, and when practiced properly, can awaken in you all the qualities like compassion, peace, and knowledge.

Throughout your day, be aware of sensations, whether caused by your breath, or any other activity like walking, showering, or eating.

STEP TEN

Sharing Goodwill

"I think this program makes the world look beautiful and more peaceful. I would like to continue." —Mark Age 9

YOUR PRACTICE SESSION - STEP TEN (60 Minutes)

This is your final breath awareness session. Even after practicing for only a short time, you have probably experienced positive changes in your psychological and physiological health, and gained insight into yourself. Now that you are established in the practice, you may wonder if breath awareness is all that you will need.

There are many wonderful methods, exercises, programs, techniques, and spiritual practices that can help a person achieve peace, health, and happiness. Each of us walks a unique path with unique needs and aspirations. You alone will determine which path suits you best. Breath awareness is very helpful and may stand alone in the way it can purify and calm the mind. Breath awareness could be practiced everyday for one's entire lifetime and continue to facilitate ever-deepening and enlightening experiences.

As I have experienced wonderful benefits from doing several of the other awareness techniques described in chapter nine, such as the part-by-part body examination, I would recommend these methods as well.

Nevertheless, for centuries, people have used breath awareness exclusively. Only you will be able to answer the questions: *Do I need more? Should I try other techniques? Is breath awareness restrictive? Will other sensation awareness and mindfulness techniques also be helpful?* If you have experienced positive changes in yourself, you may choose to continue, at least until you find something better. If you continue, proceed with utmost confidence; the secret to success in any mind-developing technique is dedicated daily practice.

It is, however, unwise to accept the information written in this book as true without experiencing it for yourself. You must also cross-examine your knowledge by asking questions, comparing results, reading books, and listening to others. If you determine that benefits are not forthcoming, and despite trying, you do not notice any transformation, then find a different practice that does work for you.

There are countless effective mind-strengthening techniques available. However, to progress in any one of them, a person needs to give them a fair trial. This means to choose one, practice correctly, and give it time. When it comes to transformation and the development of mind, positive effects are cumulative.

Your Practice Session – Step Ten

Begin with a calm and quiet mind. Set all your concerns and worries aside and know that you will be better equipped to deal with issues after sitting. Resume an erect position, close your eyes, and direct your entire attention to your natural respiration. For a few minutes, feel the breath inside your nose. Feel its warmth and coolness; stinging or itchiness.

When you have examined the breath inside your nose, shift your attention and fix it on the small area at the entrance of your nose. For a few minutes, feel the breath's subtle touch. Note if the breath is coming in the left or right nostril, or both. Feel the temperature as you breathe in; feel it when you breathe out.

Notice if your natural breathing is deep, long, short, fast, soft, or hard. When your mind becomes still and your attention is sharp, narrow your focus to a pinprick directly below the entrance of your nostrils. For several minutes, keep your focus exclusively fixed on this spot and note your concentration getting stronger.

Observe the three stages of breath experience. Note when the in-breath first makes contact with the skin. Note the touch of the incoming breath as it passes over this area. Note when the incoming breath ceases to cause a sensation. Examine the outgoing breath in the same manner, detecting its beginning, middle, and end. Then penetrate attention to feel sensation on this tiny area. For a few minutes, observe manifesting sensations, vibrations, throbbing, pulsating, heat or coolness.

Stay focused on one sensation for the entire time it is happening. When it dissolves and disappears, observe the next arising sensation in the same manner. Whatever method you choose to examine your mental and physical structure, always keep in mind the transient and changing nature of mind, matter, and energy.

Whatever sensation you experience, understand that its true nature is to arise, stay awhile, and pass on. Every minute that you are mindful and accepting of change, equanimity is being established. When the hour is over, you can relax and spend a few minutes sharing goodwill and directing kind thoughts to all the people you care about, and all beings and creatures in the world.

Step Ten is important because you will be learning how to practice *sharing goodwill*, also known as *metta* or loving-kindness meditation. Sharing goodwill is different from breath awareness in that you use your imagination, intellect, and words, and direct your thoughts externally toward others. The ideal time for sharing goodwill is after a sitting session when you feel happy and peaceful. Nevertheless, wishing others to share your happiness can happen spontaneously, anytime, anywhere.

To perform sharing after your sitting, reposition yourself so you are comfortable. There is no benefit to bearing pain or discomfort while sharing; your mind will lack volition and happiness if it is preoccupied with physical or mental agitation.

Begin by wishing yourself happiness and peace, then share goodwill with people you know and love dearly. Continue sending out thoughts of love and kindness to your friends, community, country, and the whole world including its living creatures. If you feel forgiving, forgive people who have hurt you, as they, too, need compassion and understanding. If you have hurt someone, ask his or her forgiveness for your unwholesome actions.

Continue practicing breath awareness for the rest of your life. The more you do, the better you will feel. Breath awareness enhances all areas of your life. If you write, you will become a better writer. If you teach, you will become a more effective teacher. If you are a parent, you will inspire your children to be healthy, strong, and independent. If you are an artist, your work will express depth, beauty, and truth. If you ever forget to practice, just continue where you left off. Developing mental faculties is cumulative—every minute that you practice, your attention grows stronger, your mind becomes purer, and you become a happier person.

TEACHER TIPS

And in the end, the love you get is equal to the love you give. —John Lennon

The Power of Selfless Sharing

By Step Ten, children will be confidently practicing breath awareness and will already notice slight changes in their habits and behaviors. They will understand how to master restlessness, train their concentration, and refrain from blindly reacting to unpleasant or uncomfortable sensations. Most children will feel happier and possess the positive qualities of mind that are essential for *sharing goodwill*, the final and most important aspect of the breath awareness technique.

Having worked seriously, students will feel more calm, happy, and peaceful. They may have grown more sensitive to other people, animals, and nature, and may be writing about helping the planet, protecting the forests, rescuing animals, or stopping wars. These are indications of their growing volition to help those who suffer. Kind volition and selflessness come naturally to those who practice breath awareness regularly.

For the past nine sessions, your students have worked diligently to rid their minds of harmful seeds and cultivate wholesome qualities like focus, kindness, patience, and love. Now that they feel happy, it is natural for them to want others to be happy. This desire arises out of a calm mind, which is free from restlessness, agitation, and discontentment. When negativity is gone, healthy energy bubbles up, flows over, and positively affects those around us. When we consciously share our wholesome vibrations with others, we benefit too. Sending out happy thoughts ultimately returns happiness our way. Neuroscientific research has measured elevated feel-good hormones like dopamine in people who volunteer or do community work. As well, they found that caring boosts the immune system, which promotes health. Instinctively, we know that our survival is contingent on the well-being of others. If we help people feel safe, loved, and happy, they will in turn, help us feel the same. Ultimately, loving-kindness contributes to the sense of unity and peace among people.

Sharing goodwill is the secret ingredient of the breath awareness technique that ensures lasting results. Sharing is an invaluable practice, best performed at the end of a person's breath awareness session. If you are teaching a Mindmastery program, even if it is a condensed course of a day or two, Step Ten—Sharing Goodwill, should always be the concluding lesson.

Our Happiness Depends on the Happiness of Others

Whether you were conscious of it or not, you have been sharing goodwill ever since you started learning breath awareness. When you felt compelled to help children, your motivation was rooted in pure volition. While preparing, planning, and informing parents and children about Mindmastery, you were sharing your wisdom and happiness. When you started instructing, you patiently ensured that every child understood the technique, practiced correctly, and enjoyed a fun and meaningful experience. Even if you were not consciously sending out loving kindness, you did so with your thoughts, words, and actions. Pure, well-meaning volition carries great transformative power for both you and for others.

The beauty of sharing your merits is that you do not have to *do* anything. You do not have to deliver a speech, donate money, or perform a noble or selfless deed; you end up sharing simply through cultivating your own peace and happiness. Alone, your inner tranquility, equanimity, and life wisdom radiate vibrations that positively affect those around you.

Sharing goodwill is quite a different practice from doing breath awareness. Breath awareness requires one to direct attention to the breath and refrain from speaking, imagining, and thinking. To share goodwill, you use your imagination, direct your energy externally, formulate thoughts, and think about people. You imagine the smiling faces of family, friends, strangers, and your community. You send out loving-kindness to all the living creatures of the world. You speak, either silently in your mind or in a quiet whisper, wishing all beings to share your happiness. Share your peace. And share your goodwill.

STUDENT INSTRUCTIONS - STEP TEN

Sharing Goodwill

Welcome to your tenth session of Mindmastery. You have all worked seriously and indeed gained insight, knowledge, and wisdom. Your minds have become alert and attentive and you feel calm and under control. Your self-discipline and determination have grown strong and you can sit for long stretches without reacting to unpleasant sensations.

One of the most valuable qualities that you have been developing is equanimity. Equanimity is the ability to stay balanced in the face of life's difficulties, disappointments, pain, and sorrow. Perhaps you recently experienced something sad, like your best friend moving away; failing an important exam; or your beloved dog dying. Maybe your parents separated, or you were told that you have a serious disease. Maybe a family member, who you loved dearly, just passed away. These are distressing and unfortunate events, but they happen and will keep happening. One of the best ways to deal with life's ups and downs is to be balanced. This is why practicing breath awareness daily will help you when life gets tough. It trains your mind to be calm, despite pain. It helps you observe sad or angry thoughts more objectively. It helps cultivate equanimity, enabling you to manage life's sorrows and storms.

Another skill that you have been developing is concentration. Focus and concentration help you finish tasks, learn better, understand difficult problems, meet challenges, achieve goals, and do well in almost everything you choose to do. You also have gained self-knowledge—the kind of knowledge that you cannot learn from reading a textbook or from listening to your teachers, parents, or psychologists. It is the most valuable knowledge that can only be gained through your own experiences.

You have learned mindmastery and know how to focus your attention to reduce restlessness and boredom. You know how thoughts influence sensations and emotions, and how emotions in turn, influence thoughts. You know how sensory stimuli like color, sound, light, images, smells, and tastes enter your body through the senses. You know how these vibrations affect the brain and trigger the flow of natural chemicals. You know how these chemicals can make you feel pleasant and happy, or irritated and stressed. You know how to control thoughts from jumping around. You also understand how cravings and addictions begin with unconscious attachment to pleasant sensations.

Now that you have developed many good qualities and acquired so much wisdom, you are ready to practice the fourth component of breath awareness called sharing goodwill. You will learn how to send out healing energy and kind thoughts so that other people, around the world, can share your joy. Before we learn this important lesson, let us practice a few minutes of breath awareness.

STUDENT PRACTICE SESSION - SHARING GOODWILL

Five-minute Breath Awareness Practice
Sit erect, keep your eyes closed and hands folded in your lap. Focus your entire attention on your incoming and outgoing breath. Do not miss one single breath. Continue focusing in this way for five minutes.

Sharing Goodwill
You may now open your eyes or keep them closed while we practice sharing goodwill. If you are calm and happy, then you are ready to send others loving-kindness. If you feel agitated, it would be better to do a few more minutes of breath awareness. Let us use this time to learn how to share goodwill. To start, you may sit comfortably; there is no need to bear any discomfort or pain. Sharing is different from breath awareness in that you will be using your imagination, thinking about people, and wishing them happiness and peace.

Begin sharing goodwill with yourself. This may sound selfish, but your happiness is important as well. How can you be of service to the world if you forget your own happiness? Think about how beautiful, sensitive, and loving you are. Shower yourself with forgiveness, peace, love, and joy. Feel immersed in your own healing energy and smile. When you love yourself, insecurity, self-doubt, and discontent vanish. Imagine yourself as a perfect and beautiful human being, capable of loving and worthy of being loved. When your heart overflows with such feelings, you are ready to share.

Imagine the smiling face of the person who you love and respect. It might be your parent, teacher, a kind stranger, or an old friend. Shower this person with kind thoughts so he or she may share your peace and happiness. Wish this person freedom from pain, loneliness, suffering, and sadness. Then, imagine the next important people in your life, perhaps your sister, brother, friend, or grandparent. Share your feelings of love and kindness with them.

After sharing goodwill with people you know, imagine people who you don't know. They might live in a foreign country, in a war zone, or may be suffering a natural disaster, flood, or famine. You may remember faces of missing children or teenagers who you heard about or saw in the news. Send loving kindness to these people. Expand your sharing to include every person in your neighborhood, town, and country. Then embrace the whole world, including all its living creatures; insects, fish, birds, and animals.

If you feel forgiveness in your heart, forgive people who may have hurt you in the past or who are hurting you now. Forgive them for what they have done and send them understanding and kindness. All people, weak or strong, rich or poor, ignorant or wise, need love. Here are some thoughts you may use for sharing goodwill. You may whisper your thoughts or silently say them in your mind.

> May I be peaceful, happy, and grow in wisdom.
> May my Mom, Dad, and whole family share my happiness.
> May my teachers, friends, and people of the world share my peace.
> May all who suffer, feel lonely or afraid share my tranquility.
> I forgive the people who have knowingly or unknowingly, hurt me with harsh words or thoughtless actions. May they share my peace.
> I ask forgiveness from the people and living creatures I have harmed, knowingly or unknowingly. May they share my joy.
> May all beings throughout the world enjoy peace, love, and happiness.

Thank you for letting me teach you breath awareness. May your life journey be one filled with an abundance of joy, calmness, wisdom, happiness.

CHECK-IN

- Are you more accepting of both the pleasant and the unpleasant circumstances in your life?

- Do you feel overwhelmed with gratitude and feel more humility, tenderness, and understanding?

- Do you find yourself sharing your good energy with others?

- Is your practice positively affecting your children, work, and relationships?

- When someone is criticizing or complaining, do you listen and empathize with the person's pain or concerns? Do you send this person kind thoughts?

- Do you feel forgiveness for those who have hurt you?

- Do you feel tolerance toward people who seem lost, confused, irresponsible, weak, or unhappy?

- Do you feel physically healthier? Do you feel more respect for your amazing body—the miraculous physical structure with its sensations that provide you with a way to realize freedom?

- Are you determined to continue investigating your inner reality of mind and matter and ultimately free yourself from conditioning so you can enjoy a life full of wisdom, peace, and joy?

Continuation of Practice Tip: Now that you are established in breath awareness, you may enjoy sitting with other people. Sitting with a group helps you progress, stay motivated, and keep up your daily practice. If you sit with others who perform different techniques, be open-minded, but remember that mixing techniques may compromise the results. If you are curious about what other people are doing, learn their techniques properly. However, mixing techniques is not advisable. In order to deepen your experience, you may want to attend a meditation retreat that teaches breath awareness and sensation awareness.

POST-STEPS

Post-step I - Breath Awareness for Life

Post-step II - Healthy Body - Healthy Mind

"Each time I sit and practice watching my breath, I feel more empowered and confident—no longer afraid of being controlled by the function, or malfunction of my body and brain." —*Katy, Age 54*

POST-STEPS

Concluding a Mindmastery Program

Post-step I *Breath Awareness for Life* and Post-step II *Healthy Body - Healthy Mind* are information sessions for students that can be used to conclude a Mindmastery program. It is important that children leave knowing how to integrate what they have learned about breath awareness into their daily lives.

These talks also provide general knowledge about choosing a healthier lifestyle. Although breath awareness is not about changing one's diet or starting a fitness regime, it helps to know how lifestyle can affect one's physical and emotional well-being, while promoting brain development. Even if children do not start a healthy regime when they return home, if they continue practicing breath awareness, they will naturally start making healthier choices.

STUDENT INSTRUCTIONS - POST-STEP I

Breath Awareness for Life

Welcome to the final session of the Mindmastery Program. Before we conclude the program, it is important to mention how you can continue to practice breath awareness at home. You have had a valuable opportunity to learn breath awareness, but unless you continue working, you cannot benefit from what you have learned. The ten sessions have taught you the technique and now we will discuss ways that you can continue practicing it for the rest of your life.

You may feel sad that Mindmastery is over. You have all shared difficulties and enjoyed similar experiences. It has been a lot of fun. Most of you enjoyed learning the technique, listening to stories, writing in your journals, and talking together. Even though you may feel a little disappointed that things are ending, you can actually be really happy.

Today is not the end, but the beginning of a bright and joyful future. With all the wisdom and knowledge you gained through your own work and experiences, you now have the mental power and intelligent insight to lead a wholesome life. This does not mean life will be easy and smooth all the time. There will be times when things are difficult, frustrating, confusing, painful, disappointing, and even heartbreaking. You will face many struggles and many obstacles. However, with your new skills and wisdom, you can march boldly ahead and face life's storms and challenges with a balanced and peaceful mind.

You have acquired one of the most valuable life skills—breath awareness. If you continue practicing, you will find that problems become easier to solve. If something makes you unhappy, you will know how to observe it, remain calm, and without reacting, decide on the best solution. You know that all things, all thoughts, all feelings, and all difficulties, will change. This is the law of nature—the law of impermanence.

The key to success is to practice breath awareness every day. No matter if life is fantastic or disappointing, remember that you have a good friend—your breath. Even if you forget to practice, do not worry. When you do remember, simply start observing your breath as you have learned in these Mindmastery sessions.

With a friend like breath by your side, you can courageously confront life's painful or disappointing events with a smile. When emotional storms rage, or you feel lonely and defeated, acknowledge that, *These painful moments will also change.* When someone is cruel or hurts you, smile and acknowledge, *This too will change.* When you have tried your best but fail at achieving your goal, acknowledge, *This too will change.*

Life is like a roller coaster. One day you are up and things are fun and fabulous; the next day you are low and feel disappointed or sad. The secret to enjoying life and feeling happy is to know that no matter what obstacles arise, no matter what ups and downs you experience, your mind will always be peaceful. Let nothing and no one disturb your peace of mind. Be a light shining on your path. Your own wisdom, your own light will lead you through the darkness toward more happiness.

If you have experienced any one of the following changes, it indicates that you are indeed becoming the master of your mind. It shows that you have developed more self-discipline, kindness, honesty, selflessness, and empathy.

Positive Changes You May Have Noticed

- You hesitated a few seconds before reacting to a situation.
- You reacted with kindness and understanding rather than with anger or confusion.
- You blurted out something unkind, but apologized right away.
- You encountered someone you do not like, but did not feel aggressive or agitated.
- You felt peaceful for no apparent reason.
- You listened to a friend in need and offered support.
- You were interested in what your teacher was explaining.
- It was easier to do math problems.
- You started a journal or began to write poetry.
- Your handwriting improved.
- You wrote a clear and coherent English essay.
- You enjoyed painting and drawing more than usual.
- You said, *No thank you, but thanks for asking,* when offered pop, chips, candy, or alcohol.
- You felt agitated while playing a computer game and decided to do some journal writing or drawing instead.
- You carefully caught a bug, wasp, or spider and put it outside.
- You took a smaller portion of something you love to eat.
- You started watching your breath before an exam.

Daily Practice is the Secret to Success!

Even if you cannot sit for thirty minutes, do at least five minutes. The more you practice, the more you will water the beautiful seeds inside you; your wholesome qualities of kindness, patience, wisdom, selflessness, intelligence, and peace. The secret is to practice every day.

Set Up Your Space with a Cushion and a Quiet Clock

Practice requires strong determination. You can begin tonight when you are at home. Find a quiet corner. Use a cushion, shawl, or blanket to make sitting comfortable. Set up a clock. Decide in advance the length of time that you will sit. Keep in mind that it is better to commit to sitting for five minutes than to commit to thirty minutes, but give up at twenty minutes. You have your whole life to work up to an hour! Choose how long you want to sit. Practice breath awareness exactly as you have learned. When you lose your focus, simply refocus on your breath, and start again.

You Can Always Start Again

If you forget to practice you can always begin again. If you are lying in bed and realize that you have not practiced, do breath awareness while lying down. It is better if you sit erect on a cushion or in a chair, but practicing while lying down is better than not at all. If a month passes and you realize that you have not practiced, just start again.

You can practice while eating breakfast, walking to school, riding the bus, jogging, or while waiting before an exam. If something bad happens, practice breath awareness to calm your mind. If you cannot fall asleep, a few minutes of breath awareness will help. Whenever it is and wherever you are, you can always feel your breath. If you are confused and have to make an important decision or deal with family problems, direct your attention to your breath.

Sometimes you might get discouraged. Maybe no one else cares about what you are doing or even understands breath awareness. You may feel as though no one supports or understands you. This may make you feel lonely because secretly, you may want your family or friends to practice too. When you feel these emotions and are thinking these thoughts, acknowledge the feelings. You do not have to suppress them. Once you acknowledge your disappointment or loneliness, go back to practicing what you have learned.

Be strong and walk alone. Although you may feel disheartened, keep practicing. One day your family and friends will notice how strong and joyous you have become. They will see how you make wholesome choices. They may start asking questions and may want to learn what you know. When they ask, you can help. However, until this happens, be courageous, walk boldly, and keep on practicing.

Recognize Your Obstacles

There will always be obstacles. Even your closest friends may tempt you away from practicing breath awareness. They might say, *Boy are you weird for watching your breath. Why are you trying to be so good? Let's smoke or try this cool drug. How about we get drunk? Let's just take this, even though it doesn't belong to us.* When people are bored or unhappy these actions offer excitement and are a way to get attention.

The problem is that those actions will agitate your mind and you will not be able to focus well. If you cannot focus, your mind will remain weak and vulnerable. A strong mind is the most valuable asset you will ever possess, so learn how to say no to performing actions that ultimately agitate your mind and prevent you from focusing.

People who feel restless and unhappy want others also to feel unhappy because they do not want to be alone with their suffering. When you are around someone who is vindictive or mean, recognize that he or she is unhappy, and protect yourself from his or her unwholesome vibrations. After you sit, send thoughts of kindness and love to them. Be confident that your wisdom will inspire others.

In the beginning, being around angry or self-centered people will be difficult. When you first start on this path, you must protect yourself. Build an imaginary fence around yourself. This does not mean that you will be keeping others out of your life, it just means that you are giving yourself time to grow stronger. You are like a young tree. Until your roots are strong, shut out unwholesome comments. When people are negative, merely try to listen calmly to what they are saying. Minimize your impulsive reactions; maximize your wholesome actions.

Your biggest obstacle, however, will not be other people. Your greatest obstacle will always be your habit-mind. Your habit-mind will try to convince you to stop practicing. It will say things like, *I'm too tired to practice breath awareness. I'm too busy with homework. I can't do it. My older brother laughs at me.* Your habit-mind will always try to control you. Become the master of your mind. Become the leader of your life. Take charge today, tomorrow, and for the rest of your life.

Breath Awareness Practice Tips

1. Use strong determination and do breath awareness every day.
2. Recognize your obstacles, including doubt, fear, laziness, indifference, boredom, restlessness, insecurity, greed, and anger.
3. Build an imaginary fence around yourself until you grow strong.
4. Listen to good advice, and ignore people who put you down.

5. Live a wholesome life.
6. Be kind to animals and all living creatures.
7. Do not harm your mind with drugs, alcohol, or cigarettes.
8. Boldly walk alone; one day you will attract good companions.
9. Forgive those who have hurt you.
10. Ask forgiveness from those you have hurt.
11. Share your happiness, joy, peace, and kindness with everyone.
12. Send loving thoughts to yourself.

Follow these suggestions as best as you can. If you realize that you have strayed and wandered off the path, acknowledge, *I have become distracted*, and then start again. Breath awareness is a life-long commitment. A commitment to living a good life, a life filled with joy, peace, wisdom, and success—not only for you, but also for the rest of the world.

STUDENT INSTRUCTIONS - POST-STEP II

Healthy Body – Healthy Mind

The most essential thing in life is one's health. A healthy body is the foundation for a healthy, happy mind. When you are strong and energetic you can concentrate better and work harder, which in turn help you to achieve your goals. There are two basic rules to being healthy. One, ensure that your diet is high in nutrients and low in fat and unnatural, refined ingredients. Two, ensure that you exercise to build muscles, maintain flexibility, and enhance metabolic processes. Remember that whatever you eat, drink, and do will have either a wholesome or an unwholesome affect on building and rejuvenating your body and mind.

Since starting Mindmastery you have diligently practiced breath awareness and have strengthened your faculty of attention. As well, you have been keeping your wholesome conduct promises by making an effort not to do or say anything that harms you or others. It helps to understand that wholesome conduct also includes not harming your own body. If you succumb to your habit-mind's cravings and eat junk food, take drugs, or sit around letting your brain and muscles atrophy, you would be harming yourself. Harming yourself in this way also results in mental agitation. It will be difficult to achieve any degree of calmness, focus, or joy if you continually feel miserable and agitated. Therefore, this chapter stresses the importance of keeping yourself healthy through diet and exercise.

There are some simple secrets to taking care of your body. One of the first things to learn is how to say *no*. Your habit-mind wants everything, whether it is good for you or not. Your eyes, they say, are bigger than your stomach. This means your craving overrides common sense. Nevertheless, you are your own master; the gatekeeper of what goes into your body. Simply say no to junk food, harmful drugs, excessive alcohol, and physical laziness. This might require more effort; it might not be as much fun, but ultimately you will be rewarded with optimism, energy, and health. Because you are the primary decision-maker, be smart and choose food wisely. If you are young and do not know which foods are good and which are not, educate yourself by reading books, doing research on the Internet, or by asking questions. The unfortunate thing is that you cannot trust everything you read in magazines or see on television. Most advertising cleverly sells unwholesome, devitalized products claiming that they are healthy. When a product is associated with social acceptance, fun, sex, or great looks, as you see in soft drink or beer commercials, or if the product is colorful and sugar-coated like cereal and candy, be wary. Deception is everywhere. To make informed choices, you have to do your homework. Following are some common sense guidelines:

Choose Food in its Most Natural State

Choose fresh, natural food and avoid refined, artificial, canned, and processed products. Food which is closest to its natural state will provide your body with more life force and energy. Choose whole grains over processed grains like commercial cereals; baked or steamed potatoes over chips and French fries; brown rice over white rice; whole wheat products over ones made with white flour; raw nuts over salted or roasted varieties; salad and vegetables over pizza; fresh fruit juice over fruit-simulated juice; vegetarian protein, like beans and tofu, over meat. If you eat meat, choose non-red, organic kinds and avoid commercially processed products like hotdogs, hamburgers, fish sticks, or mysterious cold cuts.

Before you eat or drink something ask, *Is this food in its most natural, alive state? Will this food feed my cells, nourish my brain, and revitalize my body? Has this food been processed, genetically modified, hormone injected, enhanced with chemical additives, sprayed with pesticides, coated with sugar, sweetened with high-fructose corn syrup, artificially colored or flavored, radiated or devitalized? Do I want to eat this food because my habit-mind craves its taste, texture, stimulation, or sugar-high? Am I eating this food because it comforts my pain, anxiety, or depression? Am I eating to relieve boredom or frustration? Am I eating this food because I am expected to? Am I choosing this food because I saw it advertised on television?* These questions will help you make conscious choices.

Keep an Open Mind to Healthy Options

When offered a food that you have not eaten before, like black-bean stew, eggplant lasagna, nut loaf, soymilk, steamed chard, lima bean pancakes, or tofu cheesecake, observe your first reaction. If you feel aversion or disgust, examine the sensation for a second and understand that your conditioning is triggering these feelings. A conditioned mind says things like, *Yuck, this looks weird, I'm not eating this.* Instead of doing what your habit-mind wants, take a deep breath and objectively examine the new food. If you know that it is healthy, try a bite, feel the food's texture in your mouth, become aware of its taste, and simply acknowledge the experience, *This tastes bland. It is slightly bitter, sweet or savory. Its texture is smooth, coarse, crispy, or chewy.* Having made your observations, you may no longer feel aversion, and because you know that the food can help you be healthier, you may develop a taste for it.

Just as you do not let your habit-mind control *what* you eat, do not let it control *how much* you eat. Use food and eating as opportunities to develop equanimity and objective observation.

Eat a Balanced Diet from all Food Groups

To nourish, build, and maintain your body and brain you need to eat a variety of foods containing protein, carbohydrates, fats, minerals, vitamins, and water. Here are the important food groups:

Protein: Protein is necessary for the growth, maintenance, and repair of all cells. Protein is a major component of muscles, tissues, and organs, and helps with all bodily functions and processes. Protein increases energy and stamina; helps build anti-bodies to prevent illness; and keeps bones, nails, skin and hair healthy. Good sources of protein include eggs, whey, soya products (tofu and soya milk), sunflower and pumpkin seeds, almonds, cashews, walnuts, macadamias, and nut butters. You will find protein in cheese, cow and goat's milk, beans (like chili beans or lentils), and yogurt. Even some grains, like rice and quinoa have small amounts of protein. If you eat meat, which contains complete protein, some of the best sources are fish, shellfish, and poultry, but ensure they do not have any growth hormones, antibiotics, or preservatives in them. You can get complete proteins by combining certain vegetarian foods like grains and legumes, tofu or chickpeas, and peanut butter on whole-wheat bread.

Simple and Complex Carbohydrates: Carbohydrates supply the body with nutrients and fuel. Once ingested, carbohydrates are broken down by stomach enzymes into glucose and become the body and brain's primary source of energy. Literally, every cell in your body needs glucose to survive. Simple carbohydrates, like those found in sugar and sweet food break down quickly and supply instant energy. Natural and nutritious sources include honey, agave, fruit, date, and palm sugars, and fruits like oranges, grapes, and apples. Unhealthy sources, like white sugar, are high in calories and void in nutritional value.

The best sources of carbohydrates are complex carbohydrates, which break down more gradually and supply the body with an even flow of energy, minerals, and nutrients. Sources include whole grains such as wheat, rye, millet, oats, barley, brown rice, corn, spelt, quinoa, and wheat germ. Many products like pasta and bread are made from whole grains. Other excellent sources are beans and legumes such as red and white kidney beans, chickpeas, lentils, adzuki, lima, and soya beans. Many of us already eat beans in dishes like burritos, vegetarian chili, hummus, and bean salad. Other complex carbohydrates can be found in vegetables such as carrots, beets, potatoes, squash, yams, bananas...and popcorn!

Whenever possible, use only small amounts of natural sweeteners when making desserts, pies, cakes, cookies, or energy bars. Avoid consuming denaturalized, refined sugars and sweeteners like aspartame, saccharin, and High-Fructose Corn Syrup. HFCS is widely used to sweeten junk food, soda, candy, energy drinks, and many common products sold today. HFCS is made from genetically-modified corn, causes considerably more weight gain than normal sugar, contributes to abdominal fat, increases the risk of Type 2 diabetes, and liver damage, and elevates "bad" cholesterol levels.

Eliminate the Habit-mind's Favorite Food—White Sugar

Refined white sugar and popular sweeteners like HFCS play havoc on your health. These sugars are high in calories, have zero nutritional value, and are addictive. Sugar pulls minerals from your bones, increases tooth decay, promotes obesity and diabetes, contributes to heart disease, increases the risk of cancer, and raises blood sugar. High blood sugar contributes to mood swings, hyperactive behavior, depression, and inattentiveness. Sugar consumption may trigger the overproduction of insulin causing a person to experience low blood sugar, which can then result in fatigue, weakness, depression, lethargy, and false hunger. Sugar should be consumed in moderation; however, avoiding it is difficult. Sugar and artificial sweeteners are in energy drinks, juice, colas, vitamin drinks, packaged cereal, energy bars, jam, pastry, donuts, candy, chocolate, flavored yogurt, ice cream, pudding, ketchup, chocolate milk, and just about every packaged food on the market.

Vitamins and Minerals: Vitamins and minerals nourish the body and ensure healthy blood, bones, teeth, muscles, heart, organs, nerves, and cells. The best sources are found in fruit, vegetables, grains, soya beans, tofu, legumes, and sea vegetables including kelp. Your body also needs iron and B$_{12}$, which are commonly found in meat and fish, but can also be found in vegetarian sources like eggs, milk, yogurt, miso, and Red Star yeast. Calcium, found in broccoli, sunflower seeds, tofu, yogurt, milk, and cheese is essential for bone health and growth. Other essential minerals include zinc, iodine, copper, magnesium, potassium, sodium, phosphorus, manganese, sulphur, cobolt, chlorine, and others.

Healthy Oils and Fats: Just because a food has fat or oil in it, does not mean that you should not eat it. In fact, healthy fats, like omega 3, are very important for staying fit, feeling happy, and even maintaining weight, provided they are eaten in moderation. Cold-pressed, unprocessed fat sources feed the brain and heart, prevent cancer, keep cells functioning properly, help metabolize fat and cholesterol, dissolve certain vitamins, lubricate joints, and provide muscles and the whole body with energy. Healthy oils are found in cold-pressed and non-saturated fats like olive, sunflower, flaxseed, and grape-seed oil, nuts, and avocados. Some saturated fats like butter, coconut oil are fine for your health when eaten in moderation.

Before buying any packaged food containing fat, butter, margarine, or oil, read its label. If it states that it may contain transfat or partly hydrogenated oil, it is not healthy. Partly hydrogenated means that the fat has been processed to have a longer shelf life. This is fine if the oil stays on the shelf, but not fine if you put it into your body. Avoid eating foods that are high in saturated fat as they can clog up your arteries making you susceptible to high blood pressure, heart disease, cancer, and heart attacks.

Drink Water: A body can survive without food for over two months, but only a few days without water. Blood, bones, tissue, cells, muscles, and brain are comprised of sixty to ninety percent water. Water replenishes your cells, helps with circulation, metabolizes fat, keeps your organs functioning, and helps your kidneys eliminate toxins. Drink at least six to eight glasses of clean, fresh water each day.

Reduce Salt

Excessive salt may cause hypertension, abnormal heart development, osteoporosis, kidney disorders, dehydration, edema, and electrolyte and hormone imbalances. Most natural foods contain traces of sodium (salt), so you do not have to add salt to your food. Instead, enhance flavor using herbs, pepper, garlic, kelp, mushrooms, or yeast. Eat raw nuts, rather than salted ones and choose low salt options when it comes to choosing pasta sauce, chips, tacos, cheese, pizza, and most processed or canned food. If, however, you are an endurance athlete or the weather is hot and you are sweating a lot, you need to maintain proper electrolyte levels. Choose a healthy electrolyte sodium drink but be careful using table salt or colored and artificially flavored sport drinks.

Calories In - Calories Out – Keep a Balance

A balanced diet with moderate portions is the secret to staying healthy and feeling good about yourself. It is also the secret to longevity. As everyone has a different metabolism, each person needs more of one food group and less of another. A teenager requires more carbohydrates, protein, vitamins, and minerals to promote growth. A pregnant mother needs to eat more of all the food groups to nourish her embryo. An athlete who burns thousands of calories in one competition requires more carbohydrates and protein than a sedentary person. If you are overweight and less physical, you need less sugar, fat, and carbohydrates and may need to increase your vegetable, fruit, and protein intake.

Get to know your body type, metabolism, and the number of nutritious calories your body needs to stay fit and energetic. If you consume more calories than your body burns, even from healthy food, you will store unburned calories as fat. If you are overweight, cut calories and exercise more, but always eat from all four food groups, even though your fat portions will be considerably less.

Recognize Food Addiction and Craving

Your dependency on, or addiction to, comfort food will diminish the more you practice breath awareness. Until you are practicing regularly, though, try to avoid the food you crave. Addictive foods are often sweet, starchy, or devitalized and may include chips, ice cream, pastry, chocolate, caffeinated pop, pizza, salty snacks, candy, or coffee. Ask yourself, *When I feel lonely or sad, frustrated or angry, bored or lazy, which foods do I consume? Do I prefer rich, fatty food or salty food? Do I crave caffeine? Do I eat sweets like donuts, chocolate, candy, or pastries?* Accept that you may have developed an emotional dependency on certain food and without judging yourself, start making wholesome choices that promote health and happiness.

Exercise for Fun - Exercise for Fitness

Exercise is fundamental to one's health and there is only one way to exercise—*by doing it.* Run, walk, jog, skip, swim, do push ups, sit ups, leg raises, lift weights, play ping pong, walk on a treadmill, do yoga, Tai Chi, martial arts, skate, ski, snowboard, wakeboard, hike, stretch, walk up stairs, bike, row, and play sports. Turn the music up and dance! Fill your day with energizing activities. Instead of sinking into the couch and watching television, or slumping in a chair to play computer games, have fun and exercise. Say no to a sedentary lifestyle. Exercise will give you energy, prevent your habit-mind from craving junk food, heighten your ability to concentrate, and in general make you feel alive.

Throughout your life, continue to educate yourself about nutrition. Most importantly, take care of your miraculous body and mind—the most precious gifts you have. A healthy body and mind enable you to experience joy, excitement, energy, enthusiasm, creativity, optimism, love, vitality, and spirituality. Remember three things. 1) Eat wholesome food. 2) Two, exercise daily. 3) Practice breath awareness and develop wisdom, happiness, and compassion.

YOU, THE TEACHER

One looks back with appreciation to the brilliant teachers, but with gratitude to those who touch our human feelings. The curriculum is so much necessary raw material, but warmth is the vital element for the growing plant and for the soul of the child. —Carl Jung

Ideally, children would learn breath awareness from an experienced teacher who had spent years mastering the technique. Such a teacher would establish a profound connection with each pupil and creatively adjust the teaching to suit the student's age and level of understanding. The young aspirant would take years to perfect his or her mental powers and perhaps eventually attain enlightened states. The teachings would pass down through the generations from sage to aspiring pupil.

Unfortunately, being educated in this way seldom happens in today's world. For better or worse we rarely experience the handing down of wisdom and knowledge from an enlightened person. Nevertheless, this does not mean that all is lost. We can at least try, in whatever way works, to develop the powers and faculties of a child's mind and to awaken his or her self-knowledge.

Although reading a book and following written guidelines is more difficult than learning directly from an experienced teacher, I hope that you find this book useful and can derive from it what you need to proceed with confidence. In this way, you will become the teacher and be able to help children.

Importance of Self-Examination

You may now be confident in doing breath awareness and feel inspired to teach children. Before you commence organizing a program and signing up children, however, it would be wise to examine your intentions. The following are some questions that you can ask yourself:

- Do I practice what I want to teach?
- Do I lead a wholesome and healthy life?
- Do I plan to make a profit?
- Am I thinking of ways to get donations?
- Do I feel tranquil and focused?

Examine yourself. Be aware of your talents, potential, and qualities, but understand your limitations. If you have genuine doubts or feel that you need more practice, practice is what you must do. There is no reason to rush into teaching. In fact, realizing your limitations is an important step. The solution to any limitation or self-doubt is to gain more experience through practice. You might even choose to attend breath awareness retreats to learn from an experienced teacher.

When you start teaching, you will know if you are effective by witnessing the results. If your students feel empowered and smile calmly with their newly developed mastery, you are on the right track. If your students seem confused, restless, bored, or dissatisfied, you may want to work on your own for a while longer. Be confident, practice diligently, and awaken your wisdom. When you are ready, use the suggestions in the next chapter to help you organize your own successful program.

FACILITATING A MINDMASTERY PROGRAM

Preparation - Schedules - Applications

The Mindmastery Program can be adapted to many different locations, situations, and time schedules. Mindmastery and breath awareness can be taught to a single child or to a large group. All ages benefit. Children under the age of six may not be ready for longer exercises; however, they will benefit from learning about them and practicing a few minutes. Breath awareness can provide a healthy challenge for high-potential learners, university students, and teachers. It can be conducted with patients in health clinics and hospitals, daycares, preschools, community centers, correctional institutions, prisons, places of healing, and at summer camps.

Facilitating a Program

This book aims to inspire adult learners to understand and practice the technique of breath awareness. Only by experiencing the benefits will you be equipped to help others. When you are prepared and willing to teach, this book provides a comprehensive teaching guide including all the information needed to facilitate a Mindmastery program and to teach breath awareness to children.

You are welcome to copy and use this book in your endeavors. The only request and restriction is that if you use any copied material, please offer it to others free of charge. You also have permission to adapt and revise the sample *Student Application Form* and *Letter to Parents*. Please ensure that the application form is revised and customized to cover you for any liability.

Teaching breath awareness to children is a meaningful ambition. However, sometimes our overzealousness may get the better of us. We need to be cautious, therefore, that our good intentions do not harm anyone or alter the teaching. Proper preparation, including self-examination, is essential.

The book explains how breath awareness works so you can comprehend the technique intellectually. However, real knowledge comes from experiencing inner transformation. Before proceeding, ensure that you understand each step in the book, as each one contains slight but important variations.

Introducing Mindmastery into Schools

Introducing a Mindmastery program into public schools poses several challenges. However, these challenges are well worth taking on because working in a classroom with school children produces excellent results. Perhaps the success is because children are already accustomed to their classroom and their peers, they respect school rules, and are used to their daily routines. Additionally, students generally love variety and are usually excited about participating in such a unique exercise.

Approach a school by speaking with the principal to see if he or she is receptive to the idea of Mindmastery or breath awareness. Support your proposal with written information, feedback from students who have previously participated, and any comments from parents and teachers. This information could be in the form of a handout, something the principal can take home and study.

Principals are usually open to outside professionals who offer extra-curricular programs, especially if offered free of charge. A principal's only obstacle, in fact, may be garnering the approval of parents. A principal will want parents on board and will probably suggest a presentation of the idea at a parents' night. You might offer to attend and to give a short presentation.

This opportunity will allow you to explain more about the program, how it can benefit children, what will be expected, and how breath awareness will be taught. You can revise the Student Introduction, distribute pamphlets, and talk from your own experience. Children's journal writing, artwork, and any photographs from previous courses will also be informative for parents.

Have your supporting material well organized and be prepared to answer questions. You might also quote research and current studies to augment your proposal. When you are finished, ask for a show of hands from parents who wish their children to participate. By doing this, the principal will have a chance to see their eagerness.

A parent's decision whether or not their child will participate will be based directly on the content of your presentation. Your job, therefore, is to provide information that covers what their child will be doing, all expectations, the origin of the technique, and its benefits and possible side effects. Parents will also want to know if their child will be exposed to ideas that conflict with their traditions or religious beliefs. Once parents understand that developing focus, being mindful of breathing, and following wholesome conduct does not conflict with their beliefs, they are usually happy to let their children participate. It would be safe to assume that all parents want their children to develop more concentration, to control unhealthy habits, and to calm down.

Determining the Duration of the Program

Once you have rented or secured a location, found a willing group of children, and gained the support of parents, the next step will be to determine the duration of the program. A program can be given during a period of time ranging from three to six days, two weeks, or even spread over a one-month period.

Ideally, a breath awareness or Mindmastery program would be conducted over ten or twenty days. However, benefits can come from almost any length of time. A short, intensive course could start early in the morning and end in the early evening. Multiple practice sessions in a day work well for teenagers. A short program for younger children could comprise only five steps. A one-day intensive course lets students work continuously without distraction but may require more preparation, healthy snacks, and in-between game and sport activities. The advantage of spreading the program over ten or twenty days is that students gain more understanding and can integrate the technique into their daily lives more gradually.

Whether the course is the full ten steps, or a condensed version, it is recommended that the program always conclude with Step Ten - Sharing Goodwill.

Student Introductory Talks

Before students apply to a Mindmastery program they should listen to the Student Introduction—Part I. This chapter informs students about the program, and explains the rules and expected outcomes. If they are interested after hearing the introduction, they can then listen to Student Introduction—Part II, which explains the importance of wholesome conduct. If potential students find that the program is too demanding or that they are not willing to give up some unwholesome behaviors, you will know that they are not ready to participate. It is better to know this in advance; otherwise, the experience will be counterproductive and self-defeating. You may paraphrase these two talks in your own words.

If you plan to conduct a program in a public facility, you will want students to fill out an application form that contains a parental consent form.

A child's decision to participant must be voluntary. This is an important factor to ensure a successful course. Only accept students who express genuine interest, as it would defeat the whole purpose of exercising free will if a child were pressured to join. If you are teaching your own children, they should also participate willingly. Breath awareness is simple to learn, but challenging to do. Children who join a program of their own volition are generally ready to accept the serious work.

Application, Consent and Liability Release Forms

This book provides a sample *Student Application Form* and a *Letter to Parents*. The application includes a section requesting that the parent or guardian consent to their child attending the program. It is important that parents support their child's participation with a signature. Please rewrite the liability release paragraph found in the application form and have it approved by a legal professional to ensure you and the children are covered.

If you are conducting a Mindmastery program in a school or public building, inform the principal or owner of the risks and liabilities of hosting a program. Take nothing for granted. Speak with the person in charge and ensure that there is a clear understanding between both parties. Obtain insurance coverage for unforeseen injuries to children, assisting adults and yourself.

If you conduct regular programs in your home, talk to your insurance company to ensure coverage. In addition, obtain written confirmation covering risks and liabilities. Some insurers will add a separate clause to your home insurance for a one-time event. Although extra coverage could add to the cost of a program and deter you from offering it, it is better to be safe than sorry. It is imperative to not disregard protecting yourself against unforeseen problems before conducting a program with anyone other than your own family.

The application also requests emergency contact information, and information about allergies, special diets, and medication. If possible, discuss with parents any behavioral or psychological problems that their children may have. This information will help you manage any angry outbursts or hyperactive behavior.

Finally, remember the two requirements for a successful program. One, accept only students who clearly express that they want to join. Two, only accept students whose parents have clearly expressed their support. Even by taking these precautions, however, the unexpected may still arise.

It is advisable to introduce the breath awareness technique in a way that allows parents, who may have objections, to withdraw their children in advance of or during the program. To avoid misunderstandings, ensure that you provide sufficient detail and description about what will be taking place.

Explaining Breath Awareness and Mindmastery to Parents

Before a public or community organization invites you to put on a program, they will want to be well informed. They will need to know about what students will be learning, time schedules, where the technique originates, if there are any religious affiliations connected to it, or if there are any liability concerns. They will also want to be clear about what outcomes to expect, if you will be offering regular follow-up sessions, and if children will need to practice at home.

Parents, teachers, group leaders, and school principals will also require information about you. It might be policy to request an official background or police check, to ask for references, or to provide proof that you and the children are insured while attending the program.

Although you believe that the technique is beneficial, others may not be so willing to accept only your testimony. Intelligent and discerning adults need well-documented, rational information to base their decisions on. With this need in mind, be well prepared. The more facts that you present in a clear, non-emotional way, the more parents will be confident in letting their children join. Use current research studies to augment your proposal. There exists a vast body of evidence showing that mindfulness meditation techniques, like breath awareness, can help a person

- ✓ improve focus and concentration;
- ✓ instill calmness, reduce stress, and manage anxiety;
- ✓ increase attention span and sharpen cognition;
- ✓ overcome addictions or substance abuse;
- ✓ reduce self-centeredness;
- ✓ manage physical pain;

✓ balance emotions and enhance emotional intelligence;
✓ cultivate empathy and compassion;
✓ enhance cognition, learning, and memory;
✓ relieve depression;
✓ boost the immune system and lower blood pressure;
✓ awaken self-knowledge and increase meta-cognition.

Even with supporting evidence to back your proposal, there may still be people who are reluctant to accept findings. Ultimately, breath awareness practice should speak for itself. If a parent or child is not interested or shows hesitation, there is usually a reason. There is still some apprehension surrounding these types of "new-age" mind-developing techniques. Be empathetic and avoid pushing your ideas on others. Trust that things happen when the time is right. There is no need to force anything, no matter how strongly you believe in it.

Important Reminders for Mindmastery Teachers

- Live a healthy life and practice wholesome conduct.
- Practice breath awareness daily.
- Teach breath awareness without asking for a fee.
- Find a quiet and clean space for the program.
- Choose an appropriate duration for the program.
- Be selective when asking other adults to assist you.
- Ensure that parents sign consent forms.
- Give an introductory talk to students.
- Only accept students who want to join.
- Ask students to agree to course rules.
- Provide options for students who do not participate.
- Ensure that snacks given to students are healthy.
- Know any special requirements for each student.
- Know who has allergies or behavioral problems.
- Keep the technique pure and simple.
- Do not mix breath awareness with religion or dogma.
- Become informed about the risks and liabilities of working with a single child or a group of children. Protect yourself.
- Whenever possible, attend programs that teach breath or sensation awareness (vipassana or insight meditation) to deepen your understanding and experience.

Preparing the Space

A well-prepared space enhances students' learning. Even if not an ideal room location, it can be made suitable. Students focus better when an area is clean, orderly, and uncluttered. If possible, remove distracting wall decorations and other visuals. The emptier the space, the more focused the children will be. If possible, schedule the program for a quiet day when noisy activities like sports events, meetings, or fire drills are not taking place.

If you can, teach breath awareness indoors. Even if the weather is nice and you are in the country, external distractions and sounds may distract beginner students from focusing on their breath. In addition, the breeze often makes it difficult to feel breath. However, during breaks, encourage children to go outside and play.

Maintain a comfortable temperature in the room and keep it scent-free. If you only have one room, divide the space. One side will be for breath awareness practice and teacher instructions; the other side will be for registration, group discussions, journal/art work, snacks, crafts, and other activities.

Each student should have a personal sitting cushion, which will be placed on a mat or folded blanket to protect feet and ankles from a hard floor. If children use gym mats, they should have sufficient room around them so they don't touch the person beside them. A carpeted floor is great, but students may still need cushioning under their feet. They might bring their own mats, cushions, shawls, and blankets, but have extras available. Discourage children from bringing their sleeping pillows and bedding. Public schools and community centers usually have policies preventing the spread of lice, and might require that you supply the cushions.

To make sitting easier, cushions need to be firm enough to provide back support and to keep a student elevated off the ground so his or her knees drop down slightly. Cushions can also be made by folding a blanket a few times. Meditation cushions, bean or buckwheat-filled pillows, kneeling boards, blocks of dense foam, and other sitting apparatus work as well. Cushions and mats should be as simple and uniform as possible to avoid children getting distracted with each other's innovative seating arrangements. Ultimately, the ideal cushion is the one that helps a student sit for longer periods. When practicing, position students away from walls where they might be tempted to lean back. If in a classroom, students could work at their desks.

Ideally, the room would have a dimmer switch to control lighting. If not, however, a small lamp will provide sufficient illumination while students are practicing. If it is too dark, some students may start laughing or falling asleep.

Keep cushions and shawls orderly. Remove shoes before entering the sitting space. Remind students to respect other each other's property.

Journal stations can be set up prior to the start of the program. If the stations are prepared in advance, students can go directly from their silent practice to their allocated spot and begin working with minimal distraction.

Teaching Your First Mindmastery Session

When the day arrives and all things are in place, make sure you have time to welcome each child as he or she enters the room. Remind students to turn off cell phones and put their things away. When all students have arrived, give a welcome introduction, a summary of the schedule, and explain the rules and expectations. You might use a name game to help children get to know each other.

You may assign children a place to sit, or if you are using a classroom, they can work at their desks. Most children like to sit crosslegged on the floor because this position is best for sitting longer. However, some students focus better at their desks.

Older or mature students might sit in the front rows to act as role models for younger, more restless students in the back rows. Ensure that everyone can see and hear you, the teacher. Students should face you. Sit slightly elevated so you are more visible and can see the whole group. Sitting in a circle is not recommended for breath awareness practice. When students open their eyes, they will watch others, make eye contact, or start laughing. As well, a child's restless energy will affect the students sitting opposite. When all students are facing you, they can hear and listen better and they cannot see what their neighbor is doing, which helps them focus better.

Once children are in their places, you can sit facing them, displaying correct posture. Ask the students to separate a little so they do not touch each other and remind them to remove their glasses and to ensure that their electronics are turned off and put away.

Your firm and clear directions will give children a sense of serious-ness and will instill respect for you and the teaching. Once students are settled, you can say a few things to make everyone feel relaxed and comfortable:

- Have you turned off your cell phones?
- Adjust your cushions so you can sit comfortably.
- Ensure that you are not touching your neighbor.
- Can anyone tell me why we are here?
- Why is it good to focus and calm our minds?
- What does mindmastery mean?
- How does wholesome conduct help us focus?
- I will be guiding you through the sitting sessions.
- If you are confused, please ask questions.
- We will also do some journal writing and art.

Wait until the children are sitting quietly. They need to know that noth-ing happens until everyone is still. Once they have learned the focus technique you will notice that they settle down more quickly. If you are familiar with the breath awareness technique, you can use your own words to instruct students. Sometimes you might also tell stories to il-lustrate what the children are learning. In addition, in any group dis-cussions you can ask them how they think breath awareness will help them in their daily lives.

Using a Gong or Bell
It is recommended, though not necessary, to commence and end each session with a resonating bell or gong. This sound will promote a posi-tive start to the session; a pure resonating sound vibration helps stu-dents tune in to their own body vibrations. However, if the bell or gong's ring is shrill, loud, or electronic, it is better not to use it. Harsh or artificial vibrations are a disagreeable start to a session.

Music is used in many of today's mind/body therapies with good results for relaxing the mind or stimulating the imagination. However, it is not used in breath awareness for important reasons. Music can calm, soothe, and stimulate the mind, but it distracts students from in-ner exploration. Listening to relaxing music does little to strengthen the attention muscle or to develop one-pointed focus.

Verbal Prompts

If you are teaching, you can use the verbal prompts found in the *Student Practice* sessions. Speaking occasionally during a session helps keep students alert and attentive and reminds them to refocus on their breath. Only use verbal prompting when you feel it is necessary; in fact, some sessions may not require you to say anything. As students progress, they will need less prompting.

Delivering the Lesson

Once you familiarize yourself with the *Student Instructions*, you will be able to conduct a session without reading. The written guidelines provide suggestions on what to say and will be useful for informing yourself about the technique. They provide theoretical information about what children are doing, with every practice session building on the previous one. In the first few lessons, students feel the breath in and around the nose. As the course progresses, they will be asked to narrow their focus to a spot below the entrance of the nose. If you advance too quickly, and ask students to examine a very small spot before their minds are sufficiently alert and sharp, they may be unable to feel the breath's subtle touch. Without an object to focus on, they might get restless, distracted, and give up trying.

In Any Length Program Include Step Ten - Sharing Goodwill

In the program's tenth step, students are encouraged to share their merits—the peaceful, joyful vibrations they have developed. Sharing benefits students' development. It helps dissolve selfishness and it generates good energy. If a Mindmastery program cannot be given in its entirety, always conclude with Step Ten. Even if you have completed only three sessions, remember to end with sharing goodwill.

After sharing, students can take a short break before they return for a five-minute sitting. Following, they can listen to the two post-steps called, *Breath Awareness for Life* and *Healthy Body-Healthy Mind.* When all the Mindmastery sessions and talks have ended, it may be enjoyable to host a small celebration with healthy snacks, artwork displays, and sharing stories.

SAMPLE APPLICATION FORM

Dear Future Mindmastery Student,

Thank you for your interest in the challenging, yet fun Mindmastery Program. In ten one-hour sessions, you will learn a valuable technique called *breath awareness.* Breath awareness is an effective exercise for strengthening the mind and improving focus and concentration. When you practice breath awareness, you will also be developing another skill called *mindmastery.* Mindmastery helps you control impulsive behaviors, make healthier choices, and gain knowledge about yourself.

When your mind is calm and focused and you are living a wholesome, healthy life, you will feel more energetic, motivated, caring, and happy. You will feel great about yourself and do better in school, sports, creative activities, work, and in your relationships.

To do breath awareness, you sit comfortably on a cushion on the floor or at your desk and close your eyes. Then you pay attention to your incoming and outgoing breath. Whenever your mind becomes distracted from your breath, you simply bring your attention back to feeling your respiration. Doing this trains the mind to stay focused on one thing, namely the breath, for a period of five, ten, or twenty minutes. As your concentration improves and you are less agitated, you will be able to practice longer. Focusing on your breath sounds easy, but it is actually quite challenging. You will discover that your busy thoughts keep distracting you away from your breath making you feel restless, fidgety, or bored. However, the more you try, the stronger your focus becomes, and the easier it is to do.

If you would like to join Mindmastery, please write a few paragraphs on the back of this application about why you would like to participate, and how you think learning breath awareness will help you. Before you join, you will have to agree to the following promises while attending the program:

1) I promise to listen quietly to the all the instructions.
2) I promise to respect other people's property.
3) I promise not to hurt anyone with my words or actions while attending Mindmastery.

Please fill out and sign the attached Student Application

Student Application Form for the Mindmastery Program

Start Date of the Program:

Times:

Location:

Teacher/Facilitator:

Student's Name and Age:

Parent or Guardian:

Home Contact:

Phone and E-mail:

Doctor's Name and Contact Number:

Please list any allergies, special requirements, or health concerns:

Remember:
☐ Wear comfortable clothing and bring a light shawl or blanket.
☐ Bring a firm cushion or a couple of blankets to sit on.
☐ Bring water and a healthy snack.
☐ Arrive on time.
☐ Turn cell phones off during the program.

The undersigned parent or guardian consents to their child: _____ participating in the upcoming Mindmastery Program and hereby releases the program instructor, _____ from all liability and agrees to indemnify the instructor and hold harmless the employees, assisting volunteers, representatives, and agents for any injuries that their child or children may incur, or for any loss or damage to property arising from activities in the Mindmastery Program.

Student's Signature:
Date:

Parent/Guardian's Signature:
Date:

Sample Letter to Parents and Guardians

Dear Parent or Guardian,

Your child has expressed interest in attending Mindmastery, a free program aimed at helping children develop their focus and attention skills, while learning about themselves and how their mind works. The program comprises ten one-hour sessions given over a period of two weeks. Children will be taught *breath awareness,* a simple focus-training technique that originated over 2,500 years ago and is practiced today by millions of people. Breath awareness is similar to other concentration-training methods, but is unique in that it does not use visualization, imagination, counting, breath control, or verbalization. Rather, children develop concentration by sitting quietly and focusing exclusively on their natural breathing.

Children who practice breath awareness develop greater observation and attention skills. The technique also effectively reduces stress, improves self-discipline, builds confidence, and awakens insight into the mind. Research studies indicate that practicing breath awareness a few minutes each day can improve memory, cognition, abstract thinking, creativity, and comprehension. Students who have attended the Mindmastery Program in the past have written positively about their experiences. They often commented, *It was really hard to do, but fun. I would like to keep doing it!*

Before children sign up, they listen to an explanation of breath awareness, what they can expect to achieve, and the rules of the program. Once they are informed, they may choose to participate. Mindmastery is not mandatory; only children who want to join are accepted.

Breath awareness is simple to learn but requires serious work. For this reason, students should want to participate and can only join with your written permission. Should your child want to stop at any time, we can arrange another supervised activity during the hour.

Each lesson begins with clear instructions on how to practice properly. Students then begin doing breath awareness for ten to fifteen minutes and systematically work up to about forty-five minutes. Younger groups would be sitting for up to fifteen minutes.

The program includes journal writing, art, stories, physical activities, and discussions. Before the program concludes, students are given suggestions on how they can continue practicing breath awareness at home, including some tips on healthy eating.

Your support plays an essential role in your child's success. Children may want to eat healthy food or ask for a designated place in the home to practice. Some children may not want to watch television while they are attending Mindmastery; others may try teaching the technique to siblings.

Occasionally, parents who understand the importance of focus and eating healthier might insist that their child practice breath awareness or join the Mindmastery Program. However, overzealous encouragement may backfire. Children who are given the opportunity to first experience the benefits derived from practicing breath awareness will often make healthier choices all on their own. Observe the small, but significant changes in your child's behavior, and let them know that you support their efforts.

If you would like to learn the technique and work together with your child, you might like to read, *Calm Focus Joy - The Power of Breath Awareness* by Heidi Thompson (Coldstream Books ISBN: 9780969814740).

Please call if you have any questions or concerns. If you would like your child to attend the Mindmastery Program starting on _____, ensure that he or she fills out an *Application Form* and that you also sign the release portion. There will be no charge for the ten lessons. The application lists the items that students need including a firm sitting cushion, shawl, mat or blanket, water, and a healthy snack.

We look forward to providing your child with a safe, fun, and valuable learning experience.

Sincerely yours,

STUDENT AND TEACHER EXPERIENCE

After a serious Mindmastery session, children often experience a happy outpouring of laughter, chatter, and creativity. With journaling stations set up in advance, students can go directly from doing breath awareness to writing and drawing about their experiences. Keeping a journal is not essential for learning breath awareness, although it is a valuable part of the program. It gives students time to reflect and intellectualize what they are learning, and to ask questions.

Most students are excited to write about their discoveries and to share what they have learned with their teacher or their friends. This sharing is vital to understanding the technique and to realizing that everyone is experiencing similar difficulties and rewards.

Journals also help a teacher detect any issues or problems that a child might be having. The things that a child writes will reveal whether they understand the technique, if they are having problems focusing, or if they are suffering any real physical problems.

Know your limitations when it comes to behavioral or psychological issues. If you notice anything disturbing or unexplainable, seek help. If you are conducting a program in your classroom or in a public school, consult with the principal. Together you can decide if the problem is serious and, if necessary, speak with the child's parents. It is important to use the utmost discretion in these situations because you do not want a child to lose trust or to feel ashamed about emotions he or she may be feeling.

The following pages offer numerous examples of journal writing from students and teachers who wanted to join a Mindmastery program or who were participating in one. The comments are insightful and communicate what many beginner students experience when they start practicing breath awareness. Keep in mind that children refer to both the program and the breath awareness technique as *mindmastery.*

Student and Teacher Journal Excerpts

Mindmastery is a cool subject and it is pretty hard. The first day was the easiest, not because of how short it was but because I was excited. The first day we went for three minutes. The second day for five. The third day for ten. The fourth day for fifteen. And the fifth day for twenty-three. I sit cross-legged on the floor with my hands in my lap. We are learning breath awareness because it helps us control our mind. My sit today was okay but it was kind of hard. Mindmastery helps me make good decisions and helps me control myself. —Age 10

MINDMASTERY STEP ONE: Today was a very interesting experience for me (and I'm sure for many others too!) What we did was this: we got our own pillows and listened to our breathing for first 10 minutes, then 15 minutes. It was hard to keep your mind on breathing because you would have other things on your mind. Like, "What am I doing after school today? Oh, I have to think about breathing. I can't wait till tomorrow because I get to... Oh yah, breathing!" I found it really hard to stay on track. I also found that I get fidgety, but when I try to move, I can't! If I were to give a tip to somebody on what to do on your first day of Mindmastery, I would recommend not looking at the clock. If you do, you would feel like it takes forever! If you do not look at the clock, you feel like it goes fast. Our goal for this group is to sit and listen to our breath for 45 minutes! It seems hard at first, but now that I've tried 15 minutes, I think I can do 45.

MINDMASTERY STEP TWO: Today we sat for 20 minutes. I found it really hard because of all the distractions. First, upstairs, there was thumping and you could even hear a pencil drop, and then roll! Next, there was a cart rolling down the hall and that really got on my nerves. Besides that, it went fine. I learned that my brain always jumps around. I can't listen to my breath for longer than 4 minutes.

MINDMASTERY STEP FOUR: I wasn't at the last Mindmastery session, so today was a big jump in time for me. Today we sat for forty minutes! I couldn't believe it at first, but I made it through. Next meeting is tomorrow, so it won't be a big jump. —Age 10

I found it difficult to concentrate on my breath because other things were always popping into my head and they seemed more interesting. Some things that always popped into my head were my homework or things that I would do after school, the time, or how much longer I had to sit for and wondering what everybody else was doing. I didn't notice any change right away but now that I look back there was one very important change: I paid a lot more attention in class (especially boring classes).

I used to not be able to sit through one class without doodling all over my books and writing notes. Now I can actually listen and pay attention. In the first week, I didn't see the point in this, or maybe I did but I just didn't want to do it. But after talking to the teacher, I thought about it and realized certain things about the group, like why I should stay in it and the point of it. This last week I think I've really benefited from this class. Last week I would have never even thought about wanting to do this another week, but now I might actually think about it. —*Age 12*

Today we had Mindmastery and when we were sitting it felt like one million black bulldog ants biting my neck. I also had a pain in my foot that felt like one hundred bulldog ants biting my foot. I had to concentrate quite a lot because there was someone behind me who was really restless and kept playing with her glasses and it was very annoying. Yes, I <u>do</u> want to keep doing mindmastery. —*Age 10*

This was really good for me. It helped me put everything in order. It helped me to not be confused anymore and stop eating a lot of junk food except if I need it for my low blood sugar level. I've got to keep on doing this. It helps me so much, so thank you for teaching me. I will always remember to take it with me. —*Age 8*

I'm very proud of myself this time. When I sat for the whole session it felt like ten minutes but it was forty minutes. I'm going to teach my family mindmastery. Mindmastery is fun!!! —*Age 9*

Mindmastery has helped me in my pitching skills and my hockey skills, so at home I practice breath awareness before my games and practices. Today our class sat for forty minutes. To me it felt like twenty minutes. Now, I will probably be even better at my skills in hockey and baseball. Today I had a pain in my neck but I let it be. My foot fell asleep and it felt like I didn't have any feet or legs. —*Age 10*

Breath awareness helps me to concentrate more and also helps me to master my mind. And today, we sat for 40 minutes and I kept my back straight for almost 15 minutes. Today after the 40 minute sit I felt really relaxed and comfortable. While I was sick, I decided to do breath awareness and I sat on my bed for a half an hour and then I went to sleep. I think that I will keep doing breath awareness because I think it is fun. I don't think mindmastery is boring. I plan on doing it for the rest of my life. And this is the last time our whole class will be doing mindmastery and I think that you should do this at other schools. —*Age 10*

Mindmastery helps me when I get headaches or when I get mad. Today I felt I could go longer without opening my eyes. Today my eyes got itchy because of my allergy. I felt like it was a little easier today because I was sitting at my desk. Watching my breath helps me when it is loud because I can just sit down and master my mind. Today it was hard to sit. Today we sat for a long time. I will probably do breath awareness when I'm sad or mad or when I'm bored. —*Age 10*

Throbbing in my legs. I thought it was *verrrrrrrry* easy. I also felt my eyes getting watery and wet. And for this time, for about ten seconds I could feel a very *deeeeeeep* sensation just under my nose. —*Age 9*

It was hard because I had a lot of other things on my mind. I'm more patient than I used to be and more relaxed. My most important experience was when we sat for forty minutes. I learned to be more calm. I'm really happy that I joined. I think that now that I have joined it feels like I'm a totally different person. Things don't bug me as much as they used to. I am trying to eat natural foods and I find I'm not as tired as I was. —*Age 11*

It was difficult because so many things were going on around us. Different thoughts kept popping into my mind, too. Some days, it was harder. Why? I don't know. It was easier to concentrate on whoever was speaking and I took insults more lightly. My most important experience was not watching the clock or the TV. It was hard and took a lot of self-control. Sometimes I would just imagine the clock with some odd time on it. I don't know if I could stand another week of this right now, but later this year would be great. Can we watch TV now? *Please?* Anyway thanks for teaching the course. All my friends thought this sounded crazy and boring. It sounded crazy to talk about it, too, now that I think about it. I *am* proud of sitting for 40 minutes. I met this challenge head on. —*Age 11*

I think twice about everything I do now. I try not to hurt anyone now. I think about the consequences. —*Age 8*

Today I had a good time. I had pain for a while, then it felt like it stopped but I think I was just concentrating on what I was doing, so it didn't hurt. I don't do breath awareness at home, but I think I will start now. —*Age 9*

Mindmastery helped me by making me learn how to focus on my thoughts and by telling me that I was the master of my mind and it helped me by telling me to set more goals for myself and it helped me to be more considerate. —*Age 11*

Today I had a pain in my neck but I let it be. I'm going to teach my family mindmastery. —Age 8

Mindmastery helps me when it's loud because I can just sit down and master my mind. I might use mindmastery when I am sad or mad. Mindmastery relaxed me so I could do more work. I think twice about everything I do now. —Age 9

I felt like I was spinning around. It felt like I was sitting for a long time.

—Age 10

Today I had a numb leg. Yesterday I had a numb leg. I can stay with my breath for 5 minutes. I want to keep working. —Age 9

I felt very relaxed because of my posture. I felt like sleeping because I was so relaxed. I noticed that sometimes it can be very difficult. Today I did way better than I did before. Yesterday I wasn't that relaxed. It was different because I never really felt that good about my concentration. Yes, I do want to continue working on mindmastery. —Age 12

Today mindmastery was quite hard for me, but I'm getting better. I stared at the spot on the floor, and then went back to my breath. I couldn't close my eyes very well. We did breath awareness for 25 minutes. It was tricky but I got used to it. The room was really dark. My back didn't hurt at all today, that was good for me. —Age 11

The very first time I couldn't concentrate at all. Some of it was just people moving around and whispering but most of it was sitting up straight and concentrating on my breath. I'm still not very good at concentrating but I have improved. The longest I can concentrate for is 5 minutes. When I'm really trying my stomach feels very tight and my back is killing me! Through all of this, I'm not the best concentrator, but it did help me a lot! —Age 14

Mindmastery is fun. I think it's cool. We have to sit absolutely still, close our eyes, and train our puppy in our mind. We do breath awareness because it helps us concentrate and clear our minds. I would recommend you to try this too. I even do breath awareness at home too. Sometimes it's hard for me to concentrate, but I actually think it's good for you to clear your mind every once in a while so you can become a good Mindmastery teacher too. Someday I just might be a Mindmastery teacher. Even if I don't, I could still do it at home when I grow up. I love Mindmastery. —Age 9

Once when I was doing mindmastery out of school I lost my concentration. Then I tried to get it back. But it was too hard. So I got up and I got a drink. And it worked. So then my mom came in and said, "Clayton, what are you doing?" I said, "I'm doing mindmastery, Mom." So then my brother came in and said, "What are you doing Clayton?" "Mindmastery, Aaron." So then Aaron said, "Can I try?" —*Age 9*

It was difficult to concentrate only on my breath because I have so many other important thoughts. I'm the kind of person who has to go, go, go, so I was really frustrated doing this, because I kept thinking about a million other things I should be doing. —*Age 14*

Mindmastery Day 1: I found it hard because I would get sharp shooting pain. I don't think I missed a breath. I found that I wanted to move around a little bit more and found that as soon as I was concentrating I would get thrown off course. I would like to focus more. I felt I was breathing through one side of my nose. My nose was very ticklish.

Mindmastery Day 2: I would like to keep doing it. It is very hard to break the habit. I just have to have a chocolate cake because if I said no, my mom and dad would make it even harder. I tried to get off my medication a year ago and I did get off it up until three months ago. I am off it again at home. I found it difficult because my mom wanted to plant a lot of negative seeds in me and it affected me at that point. I think if I keep doing this, for my whole life, I would understand myself and deal with the outside world. I also found the second time doing it at home, my mom would try to disturb me as I only had a few more minutes left. I find that it calms me down after a while. The third time I did it, my stomach muscles felt like they were getting stronger. I also felt my shoulder muscles getting stronger. —*Age 15*

I thought this was a neat experience. I think everybody should at least try this once. When I quit for a bit yesterday I felt like I was missing something. So when I came back I felt better. I could concentrate better than the other times. I didn't shut my eyes because I felt uncomfortable but I tried not to focus on things. So thank you for coming to our class to show us this different experience. —*Age 15*

I felt sore and sad because my cat ran away and I started to cry in the middle of Mindmastery. It was hard. We had to sit for 40 minutes. —*Age 10*

Today it was a little harder because the girl beside me fell asleep. She snored loud, but I stayed concentrated for 30 minutes out of the 40. Since we're not going to do it at school anymore, I'm going to do it at home more often. Every day for a half an hour. I think I'm doing really well. —*Age 10*

Very interesting to learn about. It's amazing how my mind was so full of ideas and thoughts but I could bring my focus back to my breath. The only negative I felt about this was how difficult (downright painful) it was to sit in a comfortable position. I haven't eaten nearly as much junk food this week as I usually would. I feel much better equipped to handle decisions with more control. Thank You! —*Age 16*

I found it helped a lot. It took away all my angry lashes at home. It also helped me eat more healthy food. I have not had pop for 5 or more days. I would like to do it more. I would like to take the day course from you. Thank you for working with us and for the cookies. —*Age 14*

Thoughts invaded my mind. Last session I was agitated on arrival because of classroom and family concerns. I found it hard to get focused. Also, I knew it was going to be a short session so I didn't have the motivation to get into it. In the beginning, I felt more centered and calmer. Didn't carry over the second week. Maybe this happened because I was being more of a teacher observing the participants in the program, rather than focusing on my own experience. My most important experience was finding calm, finding that feeling of deep concentration. —*Grades 4 & 7 Teacher*

I found it quite amazing that I am able to sit for so long and concentrate on my breath. I began to feel more in control of myself as I found that I could bring my mind back to my breath. It's interesting that you don't really know what it is you are about to learn but it just happens. I feel hope. I am going to try and condition my kids less and free them more. I also hope that this fall we will get permission from the students to do this again. It was hard work and a challenge, but I have the feeling that comes from meeting a challenge successfully." —*Grades 11 & 12 Teacher*

We have recently completed our last session of "Mindmastery," a course in developing strong attention skills. The students were taught the technique of "still sitting" and observing their breath. This exercise develops concentration, endurance, physical and mental awareness, clear thinking, focus, and commitment. The goal was to improve our ability to concentrate by observing sensations caused by the breath. Over the last two weeks, we have held ten sessions where we sat quietly, gradually increasing our still sitting time from five, to ten, to twenty, to forty-five minutes.

The experience revealed to the students how the mind jumps around when one is not concentrating. Gradually, through their effort, students mastered the ability to bring their scattered thoughts into focus by concentrating on the breath. This is an important step in gaining understanding and insight because proper concentration strengthens the mind and commitment to practice helps develop the will. It was interesting to observe the growth in the children's awareness that took place during the course. The children became aware of how their thinking works. Some became conscious of their thinking for the first time. Becoming aware of our thinking, *meta cognition*, as it is called, helps us control ourselves and our lives. We become responsible for the way we think about others and ourselves. Many students experienced an improvement in their concentration, determination, and ability to focus. They were proud of their self-control.

—*Grade 4 Teacher*

Several months ago, I was hospitalized with life-threatening high blood pressure. I had been an otherwise healthy, fit woman of 54, just hitting my stride. After surviving this frustrating life-altering episode, I looked for ways to lower my blood pressure and to reduce or eliminate medication. I tried a breath awareness workshop offered by Heidi. I never imagined that this experience would be transformational. I did not know what to expect other than that the meditation would last 45 minutes.

Sitting quietly in stillness, the miracle of my own breath gave me glimpses of a deeper quiet that, with practice, I could seek solace in. Focusing on my breath was a remarkable challenge; the slippery flow of my thoughts kept intruding. I realized that my own mind was denying me the profound stillness I could feel when I remained present with my breathing. My thoughts were, at times like dandelion parachutes, drifting on the breeze in some effortless, transient dance; at other times, like unexpected guests knocking insistently on my door.

The evening after my first experience of practicing breath awareness, my blood pressure dropped and stayed steady. Since my first session, I have practiced 25 minutes daily for 54 days. Recently I sat with a group for 70 minutes! Following this long session, my blood pressure fell again, this time significantly. Each time I sit and practice watching my breath I feel more empowered and confident—no longer afraid of being controlled by the function, or malfunction, of my body and brain. —*Age 54*

QUESTIONS AND ANSWERS

What does "natural breath" mean?

There is no mystery to natural breath. It is simply breathing the way you normally do when you are not thinking about your breath or controlling it. Of course, your breath will change depending on the activity you are engaged in. If you are running, your natural breath will be fast causing panting. If you are frightened, your natural breath may stop for a few seconds. If you are happy, your natural breath may be shallow and rhythmic. If you are sleeping, your natural breath may be barely audible.

When practicing breath awareness you never regulate or control breathing; you do not hold your breath or hyperventilate. These actions are dangerous and counterproductive to what you are learning—to observe reality as it is. When you practice breath awareness, you are like a scientist observing the ocean's currents. Would a scientist control the ocean in order to observe it? No, a scientist would simply study the ocean's currents as they naturally occur.

I feel dizzy. What should I do?

Hyperventilating can make you feel dizzy so check that you are not breathing too deeply. It is possible that you feel dizzy because of an underlying physical condition like low blood sugar, lack of oxygen, vertigo, or the flu. If you feel dizzy or faint, open your eyes and focus on your hands for a while. Closing your eyes can also make you feel like you are losing your balance. Once you feel stable, close your eyes and continue watching your breath. Breath awareness does not cause dizziness. If the feeling persists, you may need to see a physician.

I feel like I'm floating. It makes me nervous.

The feeling of floating sometimes happens when your mind is very concentrated. When the feeling occurs, open your eyes and focus for a couple of minutes on your hands or on the floor. Once you feel normal again, you can close your eyes and continue doing breath awareness. If nervousness overwhelms you, open your eyes, take a few hard breaths, then close your eyes and continue working. The physical sensation of floating or dizziness may feel interesting or enjoyable, and you might like it and not want it to stop. Craving a sensation, however, indicates that you have lost your equanimity. When you start craving a particular sensation, acknowledge that your mind is craving, and then resume focusing on your incoming and outgoing breath.

I cannot keep my eyes closed. Is there something that will help me?

Sometimes closing your eyes feels uncomfortable or you become self-conscious that other people are looking at you. You may also feel nervous or afraid. If this happens, open your eyes and focus on your hands or on the floor. Even with open eyes you can continue breath awareness. Once you feel more comfortable, close your eyes and continue.

Will breath awareness help me with math?

Yes. Daily practice of breath awareness will sharpen your attention, improve memory, enhance intellectual comprehension, and develop better listening skills. For all these reasons, one who develops the faculties of mind will have a greater capacity to solve complex equations and to understand problems. When you attend math class, your alert mind will absorb, understand, and retain what your teacher is explaining. Breath awareness also develops stronger determination and tenacity. This means that you can choose to study or to work through a mathematical problem. You will have the will power to not let boredom, restlessness, or fatigue prevent you from completing what you set out to do.

Can practicing breath awareness help me with soccer or other sports?

Yes. If you practice breath awareness daily, you will develop many skills. You will have more focus, emotional control, and endurance. These qualities will help your athletic performance. With a clear and focused mind you will think faster. When the soccer ball is approaching, you will be able to quickly assess the situation and know where to kick it. The more you experience your mind/body connection, the more you will choose to live a wholesome life. Eating a healthy diet and exercising will make you strong, energetic, and happy. Developing equanimity will make you a conscientious team player; you will stay balanced whether you win or lose the game!

I keep having sad thoughts. How do I stop them?

When we practice breath awareness, we do not try to stop or suppress our sadness. We are learning to observe these feelings. Breath awareness is all about calmly observing your reality as it is happening in the moment. When a sad memory or thought arises, acknowledge, *I am thinking about my parents, and this makes me sad.* Try to locate where your sad feelings are felt in your body. Are they in your heart? Your head? Stomach? Once you locate the sadness, examine its sensation for a minute or two. Then resume focusing on your breath.

I started to cry. Is this a sign of weakness?
No. Crying is not a sign of weakness. It is an emotional reaction—like laughing. Sometimes when you practice breath awareness you become sensitive. You might think about something sad. You may remember how someone's words hurt you. These thoughts may cause you to cry. This is OK.

Tears can also be a sign that you are becoming more sensitive to living beings and to the suffering of others. While you sit quietly you may start thinking about people who are unhappy, poor, lonely, or hungry. Sensitive caring is a beautiful quality. Acknowledge your feelings, send out thoughts of loving kindness to those people, and then go back to feeling your breath.

Sometimes the crying response can become a habit. If this is the case, we may cry whenever we hear criticism or abusive words. Instead of retaliating, we suppress our feelings, which may cause us to cry. Crying then becomes the way we deal with these emotional situations. Later when we are sitting, we might think of these hurtful words and start crying again. But if crying has become a habit, you are not free and must examine your motivation for crying. Stay perfectly calm and focus on breathing so that the emotions that caused you to cry will not continue to overwhelm you.

When I hear talking, I can't do breath awareness and I lose focus.
This is common. When you hear someone talking, especially if you want to hear what he or she is saying, it is almost impossible to continue feeling the breath because your attention cannot be in two places at once. Pay attention to the speaker if it concerns instructions, then resume watching your breath. If you hear talking in another room, use the opportunity to develop your concentration by continuing to feel your breath. No matter how quiet a room, there will always be sounds. When you strengthen your ability to focus, you will be able to stay with your breath even if an airplane is flying overhead.

I have a cold and can't breathe through my nose.
If your nose is stuffy, breathe through your mouth. You can focus on the touch of breath on your lips. However, whenever possible, keep your mouth closed and breathe through your nose.

My leg was hurting. May I move to get more comfortable?
Yes. If you are experiencing physical pain, locate the pain before you change your position. Is it in your knee? Your foot? Your back? Once you have located the pain, examine it more closely because sometimes the process of observing pain causes it to dissolve. However, if your pain is severe, change your position but stay focused on the breath. By staying focused, you will stop your normal habit of blindly reacting to pain and instead will calmly choose the best way to deal with your pain.

I hear voices in my head that won't go away.
If you hear voices in your mind and they never stop, open your eyes and focus on your hands or on the floor. This distraction may quiet the voices for a moment. Take a few hard, slightly louder breaths, and then resume normal breathing. Whenever the voices interfere with feeling the breath, opening your eyes may help get you back on track.

It is perfectly normal to hear voices in your mind because the habit-mind keeps talking and talking. However, some people hear excessive, irritating chatter and it becomes difficult to focus. For some, incessant chatter is a way to prevent feeling deeper pain or issues inside them-selves. If you have a talkative mind, simply acknowledge that the voice in your mind keeps talking. Pay little attention to what is being said and stay focused on your breath in order to diminish the chatter. Although the chatter may continue like a television droning on in a neighboring room, make a decision to ignore it while you are doing breath aware-ness.

I don't understand what we are doing.
It is essential that you understand what you are doing. First, you are developing your concentration. Your mind has the habit of jumping from thought to thought. One minute you are thinking about the past; the next you are thinking about the future. With your thoughts jumping around, you cannot develop concentration, and your mind quickly loses interest. One of the aims of practicing breath awareness is to improve concentration. If you can concentrate, you can accomplish your goals

and feel fulfilled. To develop concentration you need an object to focus on, breath being one of the best objects because it is always with you. Your breath is connected to your mind. If your mind is upset, your breath will be irregular or fast. If your mind is peaceful, your breath will be quiet and even. Therefore, to answer your question, you are improving concentration in order to examine your mind so that you can become more peaceful and happy.

My foot has fallen asleep. Shouldn't I move it?
Usually if your foot falls asleep no harm will come as you are only sitting for twenty to thirty minutes. However, if it becomes uncomfortable, first acknowledge that your foot is asleep and observe the sensation; it may be numbness or heaviness. Once you have made this observation you can change your position ever so slightly to relieve pressure. Then, notice the tingling, prickling sensation of blood rushing back to your foot. After observing the sensation for a minute, resume feeling your breath.

I took something and now I feel bad. What should I do?
If you have taken something that is not yours, give it back, apologize, and reimburse the loss if possible. We all make mistakes. The person may be angry or disappointed with you, but your honesty and willingness to make good will mend their anger. Saying sorry is a sign of maturity, and the sooner we learn to make things right by apologizing, the better things will be.

There seems to be a movie playing in my mind.
Sometimes while doing breath awareness, you start imagining scenes and characters, similar those in a movie. When this occurs, acknowledge that your mind has wandered and resume focusing on your breath. This may be difficult because your mind-movie may be exciting, funny, or dramatic. If you cannot stop thinking about it, it is because your habit-mind is enjoying the sensations that the entertaining story is producing. When you watch any movie, whether on a screen or in your mind, you are being entertained. If you are creating the movie, it is a creative act, which has merit. However, when you are imagining, you are no longer feeling your breath. If your aim is to develop one-pointed focus and investigate your reality within, then you will need to get back in touch with feeling your breath. When you get distracted, take a few hard

breaths so you can feel your breath. Once you have regained focus, resume natural breathing. Since your attention cannot be in two places at the same time, this refocusing will stop your movie. After your breath awareness session is finished, you might want to spend some time revisiting your ideas and writing down your story.

What does it mean to be in the present?

Most of the time, your mind is preoccupied with thinking. You are either thinking about the past or you are thinking about the future. Rarely is your mind fully connected and aware of your physical experience as it is happening. You become much more aware of your physical reality, however, when you have aches and pains or feel emotionally upset. But even when you are suffering, you distract yourself by thinking.

To be in the present is to feel sensation as it happens. Staying connected with feeling is difficult to do because your mind prefers thinking. Distracting yourself from feeling physical sensation has become a habit but practicing breath awareness can help you break this habit. Feeling each breath is an excellent way to train your mind to stay in the present moment. Every breath you feel is a moment you are in the *now*. Although thinking about things in the past or future is essential, it should be governed by choice, not by habit.

I feel funny sensations in my body. Should I focus on them?

Practicing breath awareness will make your mind very alert and sensitive to the point where a pin dropping to the floor will startle you. As your attention develops you will also become aware of sensation, not only on the skin below your nose, but throughout your whole body. This sensitivity shows that you are becoming fully aware of your physical reality.

Your goal is to develop concentration and equanimity. At this early stage of your development, therefore, it is better to keep your attention fixed on the small area at the entrance of your nostrils. Although you may feel sensations elsewhere on your body, do not let your attention get distracted and jump to those sensations. Whenever you remember, go back to fixing your attention on your breath. Other techniques such as sensation awareness, insight or vipassana meditation require that you are mindful of sensation throughout your entire body. In the beginning, however, it is best to become established in breath awareness. And once you have developed ample mental calm and alert attention, you might attempt the more demanding techniques. For now, when you are practicing breath awareness and notice sensations in the body, acknowledge them and then return to focusing on the breath. Later, when you understand how breath awareness works, you can practice sensation awareness as well. Both techniques complement one another and are excellent tools for examining your mind/body phenomenon and for transforming ingrained conditioning.

Do I follow the breath inside myself?

No. When practicing breath awareness properly you do not follow your breath inside your body. Entirely different techniques require you to feel or imagine the breath coming in through your nose, going to the back of your mouth, down your throat, and into your lungs and stomach. These techniques will calm your mind and develop focus and concentration, but you might not experience the same results as you would with simple breath awareness.

Remember to limit your attention to a small area below your nostrils, and keep your focus fixed on this spot the whole time. By restricting the area of focus, you will sharpen your attention. If you attempt to trace your breath from your nose through your chest to your belly, or to follow it out again, your one-pointed focus will be broken. Breath awareness requires continual mindfulness of breath. You are mindful of when you first feel the breath on your skin. Then you are mindful of the breath's flow over your skin. Then you are mindful of when the feeling of breath stops. Whether the breath is incoming or outgoing, the way to observe it is the same.

You do not follow the breath inside your body. At all times, your attention is firmly fixed on the spot below your nose. Stay aware of when your breath first touches the spot; be mindful of the breath as it flows over this spot; and be aware of when the breath is no longer felt on this spot. This process makes you aware of the beginning, middle, and end of an experience. If you practice observing in this way, you will feel calm and composed.

I can't feel the touch of my breath.

This is common. There are two reasons for not being able to feel the breath. One is that your mind is insensitive; the other is that your mind is extremely tranquil. When one first starts to practice breath awareness, feeling the air's delicate touch can be difficult because the mind is not tuned finely enough. Do not be discouraged. It is like trying to hear the nuances of a sonata after listening to heavy metal music. When you cannot feel anything, take a few hard breaths until you can feel. Once you feel your breath, however faintly, resume natural breathing. In this way your mind will become increasingly sensitive and alert. Sometimes you just have to fix your attention on the area below your nose for a time, even without feeling breath. Eventually your mind will be sharp and attentive and you will feel the breath's subtlety.

We promised not to lie, but what if telling the truth will hurt someone?
You are asking if there are times when telling a lie is justified. Yes, sometimes lying is what you have to do to save a person's life or prevent something terrible from happening. However, before you justify your lie, ask yourself, *Am I lying because I do not want my parents, teacher, or friend to be disappointed in me? Will they be more hurt when they find out I didn't tell the truth? Will lying break their trust? Am I lying to avoid punishment?* Asking these questions will help you to be honest with yourself.

Once you lie to solve problems in life, you start believing your own lies. This belief can lead to harmful consequences, so be courageous and tell the truth. As you practice breath awareness, you will find it easier to be truthful and honest.

Is sex considered unwholesome conduct?
Sex is a natural, healthy human activity and can be a profound expression of love that bonds two people. Physically and emotionally it can be a pleasurable experience, fundamental for creating children and family life. However, if you perform anything sexual that hurts either yourself or others, it becomes an unwholesome action.

If you crave sex or become obsessive in wanting to experience particular pleasurable sensations, you run the risk of developing an addiction. Addictions are harmful as they take away control and freedom and can lead to unhealthy consequences. When a person becomes obsessed with viewing or creating pornography, for example, he or she might experience social problems, relationship breakdowns, and even criminal charges. In the process of satisfying cravings, a person may end up abusing and hurting others.

Sex is instinctive and has everything to do with pleasurable sensations. If we did not like sex, our world might not populate. However, if sex is causing us to be unhappy, it is helpful to examine the source of the problem. When we practice breath awareness, we examine all sensation, including pleasant and unpleasant, sexual and non-sexual. Through objective observation, we gradually break our addiction to every kind of craving. This does not mean we will never enjoy sex; rather it means we are free from our obsession with it.

Practicing breath awareness can actually heighten and deepen the enjoyment of sexuality and lovemaking. This transition happens because one is not craving it, just experiencing it for what it is— pleasurable sensation. Equanimity toward pleasurable sensation is the secret to sexual enjoyment and to the prevention of addictions or obsessions. When we are free from craving and addiction, we can enjoy sex and our relationships in healthy, loving ways.

I heard that some breathing techniques are dangerous.
Yes, some breathing techniques can be dangerous. Even young children may experiment with the choking game where they first hyperventilate and then choke themselves to stop oxygen from flowing to the brain. This causes a temporary high or hallucination. The high, like a drug-induced state, can become addictive, and sometimes leads to unconsciousness or death. If a person only observes natural breathing, as is required when performing breath awareness, there is no danger at all. When you perform breath awareness, you do not control or regulate breathing in any way. You do not hold your breath, slow your breath, or manipulate which nostril breath flows through. You do not direct your breath to different parts of your body or consciously breathe in to the lungs, chest, or stomach. Your job is simply to observe your natural, normal, ordinary breath, as it is. The only time you control your breath is when you take a few hard breaths to combat drowsiness or to help you feel the breath's subtle touch of air on your skin.

What if I need to stop practicing and leave the room?
Before standing up and leaving, ask yourself, *Is it essential to stop my practice? Is it an emergency? Can I hang in there a little longer? Am I just restless or bored?* If it is not an emergency, try to use strong determination to keep sitting until the session ends. If you cannot wait, get up quietly and let the teacher or an adult know where you are going. If you want to leave because you do not like doing breath awareness anymore, it would be best to complete the session and then speak with your

teacher about options. If you are struggling with overwhelming rest-lessness, just open your eyes and sit quietly until the end.

Our habit-mind rebels in different ways. One reaction is simply to leave the scene. If you feel agitated or frustrated, leaving will distract you from whatever unpleasant sensation you are feeling, but it is important to recognize that walking away from unpleasant sensations may be one of your habits. Therefore, before you get up, examine the reason why you want to leave. If you determine that it is an emergency, move quietly and let the teacher know where you are going.

I keep falling asleep. The room is too warm.
When doing breath awareness, some people get sleepy. They may feel excessively tired every time they focus on their breathing. Getting drowsy can become a habit—a way of avoiding feelings of agitation, boredom, or stress. If you start nodding off, take a few harder breaths, as the oxygen will give you some energy. After taking these harder breaths, resume natural breathing. If you habitually nod off, examine your feelings. If you are indeed falling asleep to avoid discomfort, then exert more effort to stay alert. If this does not work, stand up, stretch, or get some fresh air. If the room is too warm or stuffy, ask to have the temperature adjusted and remember to wear lighter clothing next time.

Can practicing breath awareness help control my weight?
Yes. Breath awareness helps to curb unhealthy habits. Practicing strong determination increases our self-discipline and we gain control over our reactive habit-mind. Through continual observation of our breath, we develop the ability to examine sensations and feelings, which are often what trigger us to overeat. It also helps to become aware of food as you ingest it. While chewing, observe the food's taste and texture. The more you observe, the less you will blindly gulp, and the more control you will have over blind, emotionally-driven eating habits. The more con-sciously you eat, the more satisfied you will feel with smaller portions.

Breath awareness also helps you love and accept yourself for who you are. If you love yourself, there is no need to punish your body by overeating or eating unhealthy food. If you feel good about yourself there will be no pain to repress with food. Furthermore, breath aware-ness makes you more conscious of sensations in your body. This means you will be more aware of how food is affecting you while you eat; you will know when you are full.

You have been developing equanimity—the power to calmly observe without reacting. Use this ability to maintain your health and a good diet. For example, instead of mindlessly eating something because you are addicted or crave its particular sensation, choose food that promotes health. Instead of overeating because food tastes yummy, choose the quantity of food needed to replenish calories, feed cells, and maintain energy.

What are emotions and how do I deal with them?
Emotions are created by particular physiological reactions to what we hear, see, touch, think, imagine, and dream. Emotions are complex feelings like love, trust, kindness, anger, and jealousy. Upon closer examination you will see that emotions are rooted in bodily sensations. For example, the feeling of guilt connects to an uncomfortable sensation in the middle of the chest. The emotion of joy, on the other hand, may be a delicate, pleasant vibration felt in the heart and chest area or within the head.

Emotions like sadness, happiness, anger, envy, impatience, love, pity, and disappointment—are waves of a particular sensation caused by a flood of hormones that temporarily overwhelm the mind. Upon closer examination of emotion you may find that anger causes the sensations of heat, strain, tightness, or pain. You may discover that happiness is a flow of calming endorphins or warm, tingling sensations. Although we do not want to dissect emotions in this way, objective examination will help us dissipate destructive feelings like hate or anger. When you observe and examine the sensations associated with anger, anger loses its control over you.

Once you differentiate the sensations caused by different emotions you will understand emotions better. Do not get attached to a particular emotion. If you are angry, you may start fueling your anger with angry thoughts. Alternatively, if experiencing bliss, you may start conjuring up images in your mind in an effort to perpetuate blissful emotions. Perpetuating emotions will keep you trapped in emotion; you may spend your whole sitting preoccupied with reacting to sensations, rather than watching your breath.

I have practiced slow walking meditation and loved it. May I do the slow walking technique together with breath awareness?

Slow walking meditation, breath awareness, and other sensation awareness techniques are often practiced together. Slow walking with awareness is very helpful for developing mindfulness, focus, and calming the mind; it can also facilitate profound insight. Slow walking is a technique that can go hand-in-hand with breath awareness. However, if you start mixing techniques, you minimize the effects of doing breath awareness exclusively. Breath awareness demands one-pointed focus, which sharpens one's attention to such a degree that it can penetrate and examine what is happening within.

If you engage in slow walking meditation, it will calm your mind and help to develop awareness. However, if the mind stays attentive on only the more obvious sensations—legs moving, feet touching the ground, and wind blowing against the body—the mind might not develop the same degree of penetrating sharpness it needs to perform an inner examination. As well, it may keep the mind on the surface and not help to eradicate deep-rooted conditioning. To perform mind purification, the mind and body must be very still. For now, practice breath awareness without combining it with other techniques. Once you experience the pure technique you can choose whether to do slow walking meditation or any other kind of meditation. As a continuation of your breath awareness practice, you can walk mindfully, being continually aware of the breath.

My mind is so scattered, can I count my breaths to help me?

Counting each breath is a well-known technique to calm and focus the mind. If your mind is extremely restless and doing pure breath awareness is difficult, use counting to help concentrate. One method that works is to silently count *one* as you breathe in and then silently count *one* as you breathe out. Then count *two* on your next incoming breath and *two* on your outgoing breath. In this manner, silently count ten full breaths before returning back to one. Once your mind is sufficiently focused, resume feeling the breath without the aid of counting. It is best not to become dependent on counting, as it can become a distraction or mental crutch that will keep you from accessing the deeper levels of your mind.

A superficial experience such as counting lessens the chance of uprooting negative mind states, developing equanimity, and awakening insight. Not only is counting a continual distraction, but it is an intellectual pursuit, carried out by the thinking side of the brain. As you know, you are trying to stay with the feeling side of the brain, which is a difficult thing to do. If you must count to settle your mind at the beginning of a sit, limit it to a few minutes and then return to feeling the breath's touch without counting.

My body loses its sense of boundaries. What is happening?

When you are concentrating, sometimes your body feels as though it has dissolved. You may feel infinitely vast and light—like you would if you did not have a body at all. You may no longer feel any separation between your body and the rest of the space around you. This experience can be enjoyable but it can also be disconcerting if you have never experienced it. Whatever you feel, whether blissful or uncomfortable, remember, *This too will change.* In a few seconds or minutes these blissful mind states might evaporate. Do not be disappointed, just acknowledge that the blissful state is gone and then resume focusing on your breath.

After such an experience, your mind will be very still allowing deep-rooted negativity to manifest. This is good. Otherwise, your suppressed negativity, whether envy, anger, self-doubt, or fear, would remain repressed. Once negativity surfaces, you have an opportunity to stay equanimous and observe what is happening. By non-reactively observing feelings and sensations, they transform.

My body seems to dissolve and vibrating energy flows everywhere. What is happening? Is this a sign that I am progressing?

Focus, concentration, and breath awareness cause your mind to become very sensitive. A sensitive mind is like a finely-tuned instrument with the capability of detecting subtle molecular vibration and energy.

When you are focused and your mind is concentrated, you will often feel vibrations throughout your entire body. When there are no gross sensations, or heavy painful feelings, you experience your physiology as a mass of moving energy and particles. Your mind is able to feel your whole body vibrating. When you reach this stage of awareness, your mind perceives your body as a vibrating energy field rather than a solid object. This is an important stage given that our goal is to feel the whole body and mind as it is—a flowing, changing mass of subatomic particles and energy governed by an intelligent force.

I feel a sense of oneness when my sense of my body dissolves. Is this a normal experience? What is happening?

When your mind is fully concentrated and still, you may feel as though your body's solidity is dissolving. It may become difficult to distinguish separate body parts. You may feel more like a pulsating, throbbing, and changing energy field than a heavy, cumbersome, physical structure.

A pure mind is extremely sensitive. It can detect the subtlest physical vibrations including bodily chemical reactions, cellular changes, electrical currents, and nerve stimulation. As your mind develops further, you will feel subatomic particles moving rapidly throughout your entire body. You may lose your sense of boundaries and solidity. When you experience your body dissolving into energy, you gain experience and insight into your true nature.

When you experience yourself as an ever changing, transient phenomenon, your rigid self-concept begins to erode. You begin to experience the truth of who you really are, not who you think you are. This realization frees you from your identification with your ego and dissolves the belief that you are a separate and isolated entity.

Dissolving our sense of separateness and isolation leads to selflessness and unity. We realize that we are not a static concept or a fixed idea; rather we are a perpetual flow of energy, mind, and matter. This realization helps us accept life and death, and creation and dissolution, with wisdom. When we see that there is nothing concrete or everlasting to cling to, we can stop clinging and be free. Experiencing our connection to universal energy awakens a feeling of oneness and compassion, and alleviates our fear of death.

RESEARCH

*"It is fascinating to see the brain's plasticity and that, by practicing
meditation, we can play an active role in changing the brain and can
increase our well-being and quality of life."* —Britta Hölzel, PhD

Meditation refers to a family of mind-cultivation practices, many origi-
nating from ancient spiritual and healing traditions. Most techniques
involve stilling the mind and focusing attention on the breath, bodily
sensation, mind content, a word or object, or one's present state, while
being mindful and accepting of one's changing mental and physical
reality.

There are well over a hundred meditation methods practiced worldwide. Some common techniques include breath awareness (anapana),
mindfulness, visualization, vipassana, insight, loving-kindness, walking, eating, chakra, mantra meditations, and various yoga traditions.
There are also a growing number of mind/body methods that use a
combination of techniques. These therapies include Mindfulness Based
Cognitive Therapy (MBCT), Integrated Body Mind Training (IBMT),
Mindsight, and Mindfulness Based Stress Reduction (MBSR) founded
by Dr. Jon Kabat Zinn, one of the first scientists to recognize that mindfulness meditation might have healing benefits for adult patients.

Meditation, though once regarded as having cultist, mystic, or religious overtones, is rapidly becoming an accepted remedy, regardless of
an individual's personal beliefs or cultural background. A 2007 study by
the U.S. Government found that 9.4% of adults living in the United
States (over 20 million) used some form of meditation, contemplation,
prayer, or training such as yoga and Tai Chi in the year prior to the survey. Meditation, mental training, and mind/body therapies have since
gained in popularity, and the number of users worldwide is increasing
exponentially.

Due to growing empirical data supporting the physiological and psychological benefits of meditation, there is a movement to revise traditional medical prescriptions to include meditation and other alternative
therapies. An important paper by John Kapp, "Transforming Mental
Health Services by the Mass-Provision of the Mindfulness Based Cognitive Therapy Course" (http://www.sectco.org/A3B.pdf), showed evidence that MBCT could not only achieve similar results as traditional

medicine, but was much more cost-effective and produced fewer side effects. In 2004, MBCT was officially approved in Britain, giving general practitioners permission to prescribe it to people who had experienced three or more episodes of depression.

Because of the evident health benefits experienced by people who meditate, neuroscientists have been endeavoring to uncover how and why mental training affects the brain and nervous system. One important discovery has been brain neuroplasticity. Two studies, "Neurogenesis in the Adult Human Hippocamus" (Eriksson et al. 1998) and "Running Increases Cell Proliferation and Neurogenesis in Adult Mouse Gentate Gyrus" (Van Praag et al. 1999), found the brain to be a living organism that continually reshapes itself, not only in youth, but also in old age. Dr Irina Pollard, Associate Professor at Macquarie University, Sydney Australia refers to their findings in her paper "Meditation and Brain Function: A Review":

> Until fairly recently the prevailing dogma in neuroscience was that the brain contained all of its neurons at birth and their number remained unchanged by life's experiences. It was believed that the only changes that did occur over the course of one's life were alternations in the synaptic (Interneuronal) connections and accelerating cell death with aging. However, in the early 1990's prominent neuroscientists began to discover that new neurons are being generated throughout one's entire lifespan (Eriksson et al., 1998; Van Praag et al., 1999) and, contrary to popular dogma, these newly differentiated neurons are associated with new learning and memory (*Eubios Journal of Asian and International Bioethics* 14:2004;2833 http://www.unescobkk.org/fileadmin/user_upload/shs/EJAIB/EJAIB12004.pdf).

Research has found that when a person experiences intense sensory input, the experience can influence and shape brain structure, neural networks, and biochemical processes. When a person repeatedly engages a specific area of the brain, that area is likely to develop gray matter or to expand its neural network. People who have meditated for years show increased gray matter density in those areas of the brain used during meditation. Similar studies found that professional musicians had more brain development in the auditory, motor, and visual areas of their cerebral cortexes. When a person performs any exercise or activity with intensity and repetition, this act will shape the brain in various ways.

Over the past three decades, advancements in neuroscientific and neuroimaging technologies have made it possible to measure electrical activity and structural changes in the brain. Functional magnetic resonance imaging (fMRI), magnetic resonance imaging (MRI), diffusion tensor imaging, positron emission tomography (PET), and electrocardiography (ECG) are among some of the instruments and methods used for measuring neurological, cognitive, and biochemical changes associated with meditation. There is now considerable data showing how meditation and mindfulness exercises can effect change in brain wave activity, increase gray matter density, trigger activity in various brain regions, stimulate the production of neurotransmitters, boost the immune system, reduce stress hormone levels, and improve cardiovascular health.

Since the 1970's, an extensive body of research has established the efficacy of meditation to reduce symptoms of anxiety, depression, chronic pain, high blood pressure, eating disorders, and substance abuse. Empirical studies have shown that mind/body therapies can effectively reduce stress, increase alpha brain wave activity, and stimulate the production of neurotransmitters such as gamma aminobutyric acid (GABA) for stabilizing mood disorders, and dehydroepiandrosterone (DHEA), which enhances memory and well-being. Dr. Pollard further explains in "Meditation and Brain Function: A Review":

> Meditation stimulates the release of nitric oxide, which is an antagonist of the stress hormone noradrenaline released in preparation for the fight or flight response. ... Nitric oxide is also linked to the release of endorphins – our natural body opiates that counter pain and produce feelings of well-being (*Eubios Journal of Asian and International Bioethics* 14: 2004; 28-33).

Meditation can trigger and influence the restructuring of brain neural networks, stimulate brain cell production, and thicken gray matter density in areas responsible for memory, learning, cognition, and empathy. Brain networks comprise neurons that connect to form a database of encoded information that creates and influences thoughts, feelings, beliefs, reactions, emotions, and even physiological data. Stimulating the production of neurons is especially important for combating depression, stress, and anxiety disorders, three conditions that can cause neurons to die. Meditation and mental training effects change in the very structure of our brain's ingrained encoding. According to John Ratey, MD, author of *A User's Guide to the Brain*, the brain is a living organism that is continually being influenced and shaped:

> The neuron and its thousands of neighbors send out roots and branches (the axons and dendrites) in all directions, which intertwine to form an interconnected tangle with 100 trillion constantly changing connections. There are more possible ways to connect the brain's neurons than there are atoms in the universe. The connections guide our bodies and behaviors; even as every action we take physically modifies their patterns. Thanks to sharp imaging technology and some brilliant research, we now have proof that [network] development is a continuous, unending process. Axons and dendrites, and their connections, can be modified up to a point, strengthened, and perhaps even re-grown (Vintage Books, 2002, 20).

Fadel Zeidan, post-doctoral researcher at Wake Forest University, conducted a study to determine if even brief episodes of meditation could cause changes in the brain. Participants practiced Mindfulness Meditation, comparable to breath awareness, for twenty minutes a day for four days. Participants were instructed to relax with their eyes closed, and to focus on the flow of breath at the tip of their nose. If a random thought arose, they were told to passively notice, acknowledge the thought, let it go, and then refocus attention to feeling the breath. In Zeidan's report, "Mindfulness Meditation Improves Cognition: Evidence of Brief Mental Training" they summarized their findings:

> Although research has found that long-term mindfulness meditation practice promotes executive functioning and the ability to sustain attention, the effects of brief mindfulness meditation training have not been fully explored. We examined whether brief meditation training affects cognition and mood when compared to an active control group. After four sessions of either meditation training or listening to a recorded book, participants with no prior meditation experience were assessed with measures of mood, verbal fluency, visual coding, and working memory. Both interventions were effective at improving mood but only brief meditation training reduced fatigue, anxiety, and increased mindfulness. Moreover, brief mindfulness training significantly improved

visuospatial processing, working memory, and executive functioning. Our findings suggest that 4 days of meditation training can enhance the ability to sustain attention; benefits that have previously been reported with long-term meditators (Fadel, et al. *Consciousness and Cognition*, June, 2010, 597-605).

Another study by Zeidan, "Brain Mechanisms Supporting the Modulation of Pain by Mindfulness Meditation", published in *The Journal of Neuroscience*, April 6, 2011; vol. 31, found that meditation can block out pain and reduce activity in key pain-processing regions of the brain. Zeidan concluded, "This is the first study to show that only a little over an hour of meditation training can dramatically reduce both the experience of pain and pain-related brain activation."

"Mindfulness Training Changes the Brain Structure in 8 Weeks", a study conducted by Sara Lazar, PhD, Massachusetts General Hospital (MGH) Psychiatric Neuroimaging Research Program, and senior author for the study, reported:

Although the practice of meditation is associated with a sense of peacefulness and physical relaxation, practitioners have long claimed that meditation also provides cognitive and psychological benefits that persist throughout the day. This study demonstrates that changes in brain structure may underlie some of these reported improvements and that people are not just feeling better because they are spending time relaxing (*Science Daily*, 2011 [www.sciencedaily.com/releases/2011/01/1101211440007.htm]).

Britta Hölzel, PhD, research fellow at MGH and Giessen University in Germany, investigated the effects that anapana (breath awareness) and vipassana meditation had on brain activation. Her study, "Differential Engagement of Anterior Cingulate and Adjacent Medial Frontal Cortex in Adept Meditators and Non-meditators" concluded:

In summary, the present study shows that meditators have stronger activation in the rostral ACC (anterior cingulated cortex, generally involved in detecting the presence of conflicts emerging from incompatible streams of information processing) during mindfulness of breathing, compared to controls. This group difference is attributed to stronger processing of distracting events in meditators. Furthermore, meditators showed stronger activation in the dorsal MPFC (medial prefrontal cortex) than controls, suggesting that meditators are more engaged in emotional processing during meditation. Mindfulness training leads to increased activation of structures known to be relevant for attention and emotion regulation (*Neuroscience Letters*, 2007).

A further study, "Investigation of Mindfulness Meditation Practitioners with Voxel-based Morphometry", found increased gray matter density in the brain's hippocampus in adept vipassana meditators over non-meditators:

> The present study showed a distinct pattern of gray matter concentration in meditators, who spent a significant part of their lifetime training non-judgmental acceptance towards internal experiences that arise at each moment. Regular meditation practice is associated with structural differences in regions that are typically activated during meditation, such as the inferior temporal gyrus and hippocampus as well as in regions that are relevant for the task of meditation, such as the insula and orbital frontal cortex (Hölzel, *Social Cognitive and Affective Neuroscience, 2008).*

Professor Emeritus and psychologist, Michael Posner, recipient of the National Medal of Science, and Professor Yi-Yuan Tang, published their first report on Integrated Body Mind Training (IBMT) in the *Proceedings of the National Academy of Sciences* in 2007 entitled, "Short Term Meditation Training Improves Attention and Self-regulation":

> Our study found that with only five days of training, undergraduates trained with IBMT—a meditation technique, which uses relaxation, breath and body mindfulness, mental imagery, and music, showed significantly better attention, reduced stress response and higher immunoreactivity than those trained with only relaxation techniques. We concluded that meditation literally changes the way the brain works, modifying attention, including the ability to prioritize and manage tasks and goals.

Evidence is finding that mindfulness training significantly enhances brain activity, increases learning, memory, cognition and meta-cognition, balances emotions, and promotes psychological health. Seeing the benefits that children and young adults can gain, educators worldwide are incorporating attention-developing and mindfulness curriculums in high schools, colleges, and universities.

The Hawn Foundation in California was one of the first to implement mindfulness exercises in the classroom. Its founder Goldie Hawn, developed a curriculum based in cognitive neuroscience and practical mindfulness called MindUp:

> MindUp is a family of social, emotional, and attentional self-regulatory strategies and skills developed for cultivating well-being and emotional balance. Among the various MindUp skills taught to students, focused attention and nonreactive monitoring of experience from moment to moment display the potential to have a long-term impact on brain function and social and emotional behavior. ... Our program provides children with emotional and cognitive tools to help them manage emotions and behaviors, reduce stress, sharpen concentration, and increase empathy and optimism" (www.thehawnfoundation.org).

A growing number of studies are finding that children who practice meditation are cognitively sharper, have increased interpersonal skills, feel more confident, and have greater attention spans. "Toward the Integration of Meditation into Higher Education", a review prepared by Shapiro, Brown, and Astin for the Center for Contemplative Mind in Society, concluded:

> Meditation complements and enhances educational goals by helping to develop traditionally valued academic skills. Additionally, the practice of meditation can support important affective and interpersonal capacities that foster psychological well-being and the development of the "whole person." ... Mindfulness meditation may improve ability to maintain preparedness and orient attention, improve ability to process information quickly and accurately, and may have a positive impact on academic achievement (http://www.contemplativemind.org/programs/academic/Medand HigherEd.pdf).

Considering today's vast body of neuroscientific research, we might assume that we have only begun to unravel the mysteries of the mind. However, we are probably less advanced than our ancestors were in understanding how the mind works and how to use it to achieve happiness, health, and wisdom. Ancient civilizations did not possess modern technology, but they did understand the cultivation of the mind's faculties to a high degree, enabling them to perform introspective examinations. Through direct experience and heightened awareness, they were able to investigate the mind and its processes more accurately than technology can do today.

For centuries, spiritual teachers and meditation practitioners understood much of what modern scientists are discovering today. The Vedic Indian scriptures, dating back more than five thousand years, taught various forms of meditation and mind development. There are vast collections of sacred writings that explain not only how the mind works, but how a person can cultivate its potential and achieve extraordinary powers. Much of this knowledge has been forgotten, misunderstood, or dismissed as non-scientific. Society has become excessively materialistic and has invested more time in acquiring external things and intellectual and scientific knowledge, and less on developing mental powers, happiness, and wisdom. Mystics from the past often spent an entire lifetime investigating the mind's extraordinary levels of consciousness. They used the mind as a means to free themselves from ignorance and delusion, and to become enlightened.

Modern science, with its focus on external facts and data, will never prove what an individual experiences spiritually. Scientific facts may give us confidence and inspiration to proceed with our inner investigation, but they can only help us intellectually. Even scientists themselves may miss the point if they fail to use their knowledge to become healthier and happier.

No amount of research can change us—only we can change ourselves. Facts, proven in a laboratory or under a microscope, cannot free us from ignorance and suffering. There are far greater benefits to meditation than can possibly be measured through scientific technology. Experiencing your transient mind/body phenomenon, reshaping your mental structure, and purifying your subconscious are miraculous events, far beyond what science can do for you. The most important discovery of this century will happen when you embark on your inner journey and follow the road that no one else can travel or verify—a unique and personal path toward self-realization, compassion, and joy.

IN CONCLUSION

Congratulations! You have now arrived at the end of the program. With strong determination, diligent effort, and powerful concentration you have successfully worked through Mindmastery's ten steps and have acquired invaluable skills and insight through practicing breath awareness. Although this is the end, it is the beginning of a life filled with abundant focus, peace, joy, and goodwill. You have learned the amazing technique of breath awareness and through dedicated practice you have strengthened your mental faculties, learned how your mind works, and developed a most valuable quality—equanimity.

Throughout your life, you will inevitably encounter day-to-day problems, issues, upsets, disputes, and even hard-to-break habits. Nevertheless, these obstacles will be less daunting than they were before learning breath awareness. Your precious daily hour of sitting and your continual awareness of breath will be there to help you through these tougher times so you can still enjoy life. Breath awareness will always be a friend you can depend on.

You have now discovered how to transform unwholesome conditioning and unhealthy habits through the objective observation of breath and sensation. You also understand that everything, including your body and mind are in constant flux and that nothing is permanent. You realize that peace and happiness come naturally to those who stop clinging to the changing phenomenon of life.

The goal of practicing breath awareness is always the same—to develop equanimity toward whatever manifests and to establish peace and harmony within. Being balanced, despite life's unavoidable ups and downs, painful and pleasurable sensations, or successes and failures is the secret to being happy. We cannot change the world or avoid problems, but we can change our reactions toward what happens to us.

You have taken the first step on a truly wonderful path that will lead to inner peace and great wisdom. And as you continue your journey you will discover that breath awareness is a precious key. Little by little, this key will open the door to the mysterious world within you. One day you will enter its magnificent space and know who you are. Fear and self-doubt will vanish. You will feel infinitely connected with all life—a sense of unity that is the most sacred of all human feelings.

ABOUT THE AUTHOR

Heidi Thompson was born in Vernon, British Columbia, a small town in western Canada. She traveled to Switzerland in the early 1970's and trained as a photographer at the *University of Art & Design* in Zürich. Thompson then moved to Germany and continued her fine art studies at the *Akademie der Bildene Künste* in Nürnberg where she studied painting for a year before relocating to Budapest, where Thompson attended the *Hungarian Art Academy* for a year of painting. While in Europe, she became interested in psychology, yoga, mind development, and meditation. She attended retreats and workshops that taught a variety of meditation techniques.

In 1982, Thompson returned to Vernon and worked as a freelance painter and photographer, exhibiting her art in Canada and the United States. During this time, she continued to investigate various methods of meditation, which led her to attend a 10-day vipassana course taught by S.N. Goenka. This silent retreat offered a disciplined schedule of waking at four in the morning and practicing meditation for about ten hours each day. Students performed anapana (breath awareness) for three days, vipassana (sensation awareness) for the remaining seven, and concluded the program with *metta* (sharing goodwill), on day ten. In the evenings, students listened to a recorded discourse by Goenka explaining the technique and theory of vipassana. Students were provided vegetarian meals, lodging, and meditation instructions. There was no cost to join; the retreats were supported by *dana*—donations and volunteer service offered by former students. For Thompson, the experience was transformational and profoundly affected the rest of her life. Over the next twenty-eight years, she would attend vipassana courses, each time deepening her understanding about herself and the technique.

In 1984, she married Edward Thompson and a few years later gave birth to their daughter Carmen. Over the years, she would take Carmen to children's anapana courses. Thompson would participate in the programs serving as a children's counselor or course manager. In 1996, ten years after having first learned anapana, Thompson wanted to teach it to young people. Because the technique is non-religious, she believed that it would be an ideal focus-training technique for children in public schools. She created a *Mindmastery* program also called, *Advanced Attention Development* (AAD), designed specifically for young people. To the surprise of many, teachers and school principals welcomed AAD into their classrooms. This acceptance may have been partly due to the significant increase in attention deficit and hyperactivity disorders during the 1990's along with escalating behavioral problems in youth. Children of all ages and abilities participated in the AAD workshops including high-potential learners, the learning-disabled, at-risk teenagers, and children suffering attention and behavioral problems. Virtually everyone who attended enjoyed the lessons, felt that they benefited, and improved their ability to focus.

Some teachers who participated in the program recorded their students' progress. They noted significant improvements in learning, handwriting, meta-cognition, art, comprehension, and listening skills. Based on the results and observations of children who attended AAD, Thompson wrote "Teaching Children Concentration," an article that was later published in Vancouver's *Common Ground* magazine in 1999. Response to the article was overwhelming and Thompson received a flood of letters from teachers, principals, parents, doctors, psychologists, counselors, and naturopaths requesting more information. Some wanted to learn the technique to help their children, students, or patients; others asked if there were any teachers who would facilitate an AAD program in their home, school, or community. In addition, many wanted to learn breath awareness for themselves.

To be more involved in public education, Thompson returned to university in 2001 and earned her B.F.A. and then a B.C. Teaching Certificate. Teaching part-time in high schools and elementary schools gave her an insider's perspective on today's education and school culture. In her writings and articles, Thompson acknowledges the many positive factors of academic learning, along with the difficulties facing today's educators. Nevertheless, she stresses that students' learning, especially their brain development and emotional well-being, could significantly improve by incorporating additional attention development and introspective curriculums in classrooms. In 2012, Thompson wrote and published Calm Focus Joy to provide educators and parents with an aid that could be used in the home or classroom to teach breath awareness to children. She currently lives and works in Vernon, and spends her time painting, exhibiting, writing, and conducting workshops.

CPSIA information can be obtained at www.ICGtesting.com
Printed in the USA
LVOW122318220412

278522LV00003B/2/P